Inconceivable

Inconceivable

On the True Meaning of Family

REBECCA COXON

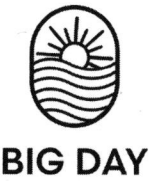

BIG DAY

Big Day
An imprint of HarperCollins*Publishers*
1 London Bridge Street
London SE1 9GF

www.bigdaybooks.co.uk

HarperCollins*Publishers*
Macken House, 39/40 Mayor Street Upper
Dublin 1, D01 C9W8, Ireland

First published in Great Britain in 2026 by 4th Estate

1

Copyright © Rebecca Coxon 2026

Rebecca Coxon asserts the moral right to be identified as the author of this work in accordance with the Copyright, Designs and Patents Act 1988

A catalogue record for this book is available from the British Library

HB ISBN 978-0-00-872635-5
TPB ISBN 978-0-00-872636-2

All rights reserved. No part of this publication may be reproduced, stored in a retrieval system, or transmitted, in any form or by any means, electronic, mechanical, photocopying, recording or otherwise, without the prior permission of the publishers.

Without limiting the exclusive rights of any author, contributor or the publisher of this publication, any unauthorised use of this publication to train generative artificial intelligence (AI) technologies is expressly prohibited. HarperCollins also exercise their rights under Article 4(3) of the Digital Single Market Directive 2019/790 and expressly reserve this publication from the text and data mining exception.

Typeset in 12.5/15.5 Dante MT Std by Six Red Marbles UK, Thetford, Norfolk

Printed and bound in [CPI Group (UK) Ltd, Croydon]

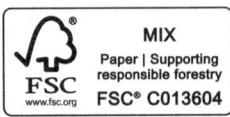

To my family,
With all my love

Contents

Family	1
Coincidence	5
Shame	23
Curious	31
Baby	40
Donor	55
Labour	59
Wanted	75
Time	88
Space	99
Tissue	108
Blood	122
Belly	129
Ghost	136
Artificial	149
Anonymous	162
Egg	176
Immaculate	183
Golden	190
Hen	206
Christmas	219
Concrete	227
Swimmers	234
Frozen	242
Patient	259
Single	270
Art	286
Half	298
Crazy	303
Story	317
Epilogue	329
Acknowledgements	339

Family

Definition

1. A group of parents and their children
2. Descendants of a common ancestor

Above my grandma's bed hung a framed black-and-white photograph of my dad. As a small child I quietly admired it; his luminous eyes, dark hair and gentle smile. He embodied a tender, yet spirited early adulthood, staring plumbly into the future. Handsome and seeking. I liked seeing him up there in pride of place – my grandma's only child – a real-life younger person, long before I was born. It gave me a comforting sense of faux-nostalgia.

A few years later, I would discover that it was not, in fact, a photograph of my dad but of a man called Elvis Presley. I was confused because he looked so similar to my dad and embarrassed because everyone else seemed to know who he was. Apparently he was very famous. My grandma had been a lifelong fan. My parents laughed; an adorable mistake, but I felt a hot pulse of humiliation. It was the first time an assumption had betrayed me.

Ten years later, over a family breakfast, it was mentioned in passing that the same grandmother was not blood-related to us. We shared her surname but not her genes. I was sipping orange juice when a swell of disorientation surged over me. It was another detail that the rest of the family apparently knew but had never told me; they thought 'I already knew'. How had this information passed me by? My siblings seemed nonplussed, which left me feeling more adrift. Something like shame squelched in my throat as I asked questions that I had never expected to ask. When did you all find out? Does that mean that none of Dad's side of the family is related to us?

The biology mattered less to me than the secret. It was the unintentional ignorance, the isolated obliviousness of it all that felt like a lump of salt in my tea; jolting me to reassess my place in the family of things, as Mary Oliver put it. I felt foolish and found myself treading more carefully from then on, not wanting to disturb the dirt too much in case any clues had been left there. Meanwhile the world goes on.

Dad had been adopted, it turned out. A classic affliction of the 1950s, in which young, unmarried couples were forced to give away their newborn babies. My grandparents adopted him, after their own tragic stillbirth, and that was that. We were not to talk about it with him. Mum warned us that she had brought it up a few times over their fifty-year marriage, but the reaction was always the same: he had no interest in finding out who his birth parents were.

'As far as he's concerned his adopted parents were his parents,' Mum told me. 'He didn't want to upset them by going looking for anyone.'

But I was always curious. I grew up, went to university and sustained a career in curiosity: making investigative documentaries for television and moonlighting as a ghostwriter. I was always asking questions, learning about the world, searching for some kind of universal truth.

The story of where my dad came from – and therefore where my siblings and I all came from – fascinated me. He was adopted, his birth parents gave him away, but it was likely they'd had no real choice. They were teenagers, apparently. They had even given him a name, Michael, which his adopted parents changed to John. Knowing that he had once had a different name felt odd and unsettling. Where did he come from?

My grandfather died before I was born and my grandmother – the one with the Elvis photo – passed away when I was eight years old, so there was no one left to ask. Dad didn't want to upset anyone, but now his parents were gone, I wondered, did he ever think about his birth family? I knew he would never go down the route of looking, but perhaps I could find out a bit more. I didn't want to track anyone down or reopen old wounds, yet I felt I had a right to know where those teenagers had come from. They were my genetic grandparents after all. Dad has an unusual combination of curly black hair, light blue eyes and easily tanned skin. Perhaps his ancestors were Irish or German or Australian, I wondered. Maybe his biological parents were still alive. They might be only fifteen or so years older than him, in their eighties now. A sense of sorrow for them lingered in my heart. Nobody forgets a baby.

Another decade passed, but my curiosity quietly remained. When I saw an advert for a DNA website called 23andMe in December 2016, I signed up to its Christmas offer straight away. It was perfect – I could discreetly find out more without needing to ask Dad. The transaction was simple: send off some saliva in the post and six weeks later the results would appear on my phone as a full genetic ancestry and personal health profile.

One day I mentioned it to Mum in passing.

'Are you sure you want to know?' she asked.

I had not told her that my purchase had been triggered by an interest in Dad's side of the family.

'Yeah, why not?' I replied.

'You might find out something you wish you didn't know.'

'But I'd rather know than not know.'

'Insurance companies could use the data against you in the future,' she warned.

It wasn't unusual for Mum to worry about such matters. Just another thing for me to roll my eyes at then forget about, along with tax returns, dentist appointments and pension plans.

'I'm not worried about that,' I said. 'It doesn't bother me.'

'Okay, well you can't go back once you find something out,' she said, in one final push.

I thought Mum was concerned about me finding a faulty gene, perhaps a predisposition to Parkinson's or a certain cancer. Maybe I was a carrier for something serious and would have to think twice about having kids. It didn't cross my mind that she might be talking about anything else.

Six weeks later, the results came back. European ancestors: 95 per cent from the United Kingdom and Ireland. Boring. I had no close DNA relatives on the site. I was slightly more prone to late-onset Alzheimer's. Oh well. I told my family at our next gathering and showed them the maps and pie charts on my phone.

'Cool,' they said, and that was it.

Three years later, I logged on to the website again, clicked on a button and everything changed.

Irony, in its broadest sense, is the juxtaposition of an expectation and an opposing reality. I had signed up to the DNA website to discover more about my dad's origins and learn more about our shared ancestry, but it revealed that he was not my biological father.

Coincidence

Definition

1. An accidental occurrence of events that happen at the same time
2. An occurrence of events that appear to be connected but are not

In March 2019, I was working on a Channel 4 documentary called *The Family Secret* when my own came to light. Sitting at a cramped desk inside a cave-like edit suite in south-west London, I was browsing the news during my lunch break when I came across an intriguing article. It was about a woman who had undergone a preventative double mastectomy at the age of twenty-three to reduce her chances of getting breast cancer later in life, after discovering she carried the BRCA1 gene. Ten years on, she learned that her test results had been incorrect and her mastectomy had been unnecessary.

I logged on to the 23andMe app to check my genetic report. I had not noticed anything about this gene on my results before, but I knew that DNA websites were constantly updating and upgrading their technology. I wanted to check for peace of mind.

I was negative for the BRCA gene, and relieved, but I noticed the tab called 'DNA relatives' had been 'updated' so I clicked on it. Previously only distant relatives – third or fourth cousins – had been listed. Now a new person had appeared right at the top.

Lucy. Half-sister. 27.9% DNA shared.

I stared at the screen. It made no sense. I didn't have a half-sister. I didn't know anyone with that surname. It must be a mistake. I googled 'Wrong DNA match'.

Very rare, 99.9% accurate, possible but unlikely.

I clicked on Lucy's profile.

Birth Year 1990. Location, England.

As an IVF child ('made' in Nottingham Queens Medical Centre, UK) I would love to find my biological dad.

We were born six months apart. I read the words again. I was even more confused. Like me, she had been conceived in Nottingham and she was an IVF child.

I had known since I was a teenager that my siblings and I were conceived by in vitro fertilisation: outside of the womb, in a Petri dish. There are four of us in total: Tim, me, Joe and Ruth, in that order. The latter three of us being born on the same day.

People are fascinated by triplets so from a young age we were used to getting questions, but no one had ever mentioned the method of our conception. Most people don't want to think about it. Like everyone else, I had just assumed it was the birds and the bees, and maybe a hiccup of Mother Nature to produce three babies at once. Then one day, when we were fourteen, we learned about IVF in a Religious Education lesson. It was mentioned that multiples were often conceived this way and someone asked if we had been. On the car ride home from school we brought it up with Mum. She was uncharacteristically quiet.

'Were *we* IVF?' Joe asked.

Mum stared ahead at the road. 'I'm not saying anything,' she replied eventually, 'because I need to talk to Dad before I answer any questions.'

My stomach dropped. She never normally needed to consult Dad.

'Were we adopted?' I asked, half-joking.

'No, no, no,' Mum said.

I was confused. If we were IVF, why didn't she just tell us? It wasn't a big deal; I thought it was pretty cool, actually.

Later I searched the internet and discovered that having triplets spontaneously (without fertility treatment) is exceptionally rare: a one in eight thousand chance. Triplets conceived with IVF, on the other hand, made up about 5 per cent of IVF births in the 1990s, so were much more common. That evening our parents admitted to us that, yes, we had been conceived with IVF.

'Why didn't you tell us before?' I asked.

'We didn't want other children at school to make you feel weird,' Mum replied, 'or like you weren't normal.'

It made sense. We didn't have a problem with it; it just became an addition to our arsenal of fun facts. Now we weren't just triplets, we were *IVF* triplets. But more than a decade later, here I was unable to understand how I could have a genetically related half-sibling. Perhaps my dad had donated some leftover sperm during the IVF process for another family to use? Or maybe there had been a mix-up in the lab? I googled 'sperm mix-up'.

Mix-ups of sperm specimens can lead to litigation for medical negligence.

I took a screenshot then wandered into my workplace's communal kitchen to microwave some pasta. A colleague asked how I was doing and I explained what had just happened.

'Oh wow,' she said. 'Imagine if the clinic messed up and it turns into a big exposé or something. You could make a documentary about it.'

The thought had already crossed my mind. The type of documentaries I worked on were all about scoops and scandals; bringing justice to light. We were always looking to develop new stories or new angles on old stories. But first I needed to find out more facts. I went outside, into the February-chilled streets, and called Mum.

'Hello darling, what's up?' she answered in her usual cheery tone. I could tell she was dog-grooming. For more than thirty years Mum has run her own dog-grooming business from the 'poodle parlour', a shed outside our house that my dad built, custom-fitted with a shower and kennels. But even if she was working, she would always answer the phone if it was one of us.

'Hello, so something really weird has just happened,' I said. 'You know I did that DNA test a while ago?'

'Yeah.'

'Well, I've just logged on and clicked on something and it says I have a half-sister.'

'What?' she said, surprised.

'Yeah. I don't really understand. It says she's on the paternal side.'

There was a long pause from both of us.

'Perhaps Dad's sperm was donated to another family as well?' I suggested, eventually. 'Did they ask you if they could do that?'

'No.'

Silence again.

'Are you there?' I asked.

'Yes, it's just that you've dropped a bit of a bombshell on me and I'm not sure what to say.'

I could feel her shock thrumming through the phone.

'Are you sure it's a half-sister?' Mum asked. 'She might be an aunt or cousin from Dad's side of the family that we don't know about, because he was adopted.'

'Yeah maybe. I'll do some more research and find out.'

We said goodbye, hung up and I got straight back on to the internet. I discovered that on average full siblings share around 50 per cent of their DNA and half-siblings share around 25 per cent. Lucy and I shared 28 per cent. Other relations that share a quarter of your DNA include a grandparent, aunt, uncle, niece or nephew. But Lucy was only six months older than me. The other possibility, the internet said, was that we were double first cousins, meaning our fathers were brothers and our mothers were sisters. It seemed wildly unlikely, but made more sense due to our similar ages.

Fifteen minutes later Mum and I continued our conversation over WhatsApp.

> Is it possible she is an aunt?

> If Dad has a brother who was a donor then yes

> Hold on. But for her to be my aunt ... She would have to be dad's sister. Full sister. Which means dad's mum and dad would have to have had another child ... and for some reason that child doesn't know who her dad is

> And there would be a 40 year gap between dad and his sister. Is that right?

> Too complicated for me!

> I know lol!

> Could she be your cousin?

> Well from what I've been reading ... our 28% match and the fact we share an X chromosome means that we are more likely to be half-siblings or aunt/niece. I think it COULD be possible we are 1st cousins, but rare.

> Btw is your payslip correct?

Mum changed the subject here, steering the conversation on to taxes and payslips, things I always ran by her. Something more tangible and easy to control. I joked that with all this distraction at work, I definitely wasn't earning my wage that day.

When I got home that evening I told my boyfriend, Sam, what

had happened. Sam and I had met three years earlier in a blues bar in east London. I was charmed by his Canadian accent and confident energy and he by my relaxed but ruminating nature. He was always immaculately groomed and had the straightest teeth I'd ever seen. He worked for an international law firm and had relocated from Toronto to London because he liked travelling and fancied a challenge and a change of scenery. We lived together in a beautiful second-floor corner flat in Shoreditch – a stone's throw from Spitalfields Market – with exposed brick walls and enormous windows. When I told him about what I'd found on the DNA website he seemed to find it all rather exciting.

'I can't wait to see how this unfolds,' he said. 'It's like I'm waiting for the next episode.'

'I know,' I said, my tummy twisting. 'It doesn't feel real.'

The scenario felt even more meta for both of us because at the time we had been binge-watching a series on Netflix called *Jane the Virgin*. The American sitcom follows a twenty-three-year-old woman called Jane who makes a vow to her religious grandmother that she will save her virginity until marriage, but in a twist of fate she becomes pregnant after an artificial insemination mix-up by her gynaecologist. Things get more awkward when it transpires not only that the sperm came from Jane's boss but that it was his last frozen semen sample after cancer treatment, so he convinces her to continue the pregnancy. Sam and I joked that we were now living in an episode of the fictional TV drama, except I wasn't Jane; I was the baby in her belly, all grown up and asking questions.

'So the only thing you know for certain,' Sam said, 'is that you share 28 per cent of your genes with this woman called Lucy?'

'Yes,' I replied.

'And the website says you share it on your father's side?'

'Yeah.'

'So you and Lucy share the same father.'

'It seems that way.'

'So either your dad is father to both of you. Or you both have a different father.'

'Oh my god,' I said. 'I hadn't thought of that.'

I had only considered that my dad's sperm had been given to another family, not that we shared a different father entirely. I started to panic. How had something so obvious eluded me? I felt sick and immobilised. I decided to message Lucy on the website.

> Hi Lucy, hope you're well. This DNA result comes as a bit of a surprise! I think it's possible we could also be 1st cousins or aunt/niece, so it would be good to swap more information. Can I ask what you know about your biological dad?

Lucy replied swiftly.

> Hello! My dad was a sperm donor, I was made in Nottingham Queens Medical Centre and born in 1990. As far as I know they tried to match my dad (the man who raised me) to the donor so apparently he was a young medical student, 6 foot 3 with green eyes. Not sure how true that is but my twin sister (not identical) and I are both green grey eyes and 5 foot 8ish. Amazing to have a new blood relative! Was your dad a sperm donor? I'd love to hear more. Thank you for getting in touch :)

I screengrabbed the message and sent it to Mum.

> This is so confusing. So now I'm worried that the young medical student's sperm got mixed up with dad's. Or that's just a made up story.
>
>   Or . . . am I not related to dad?

Two blue ticks. Mum had read the messages. Four minutes passed.

Lol you ok? You there?

Talking to Dad now. He doesn't know about Lucy (he's been at work and in the bath). It'll take a while to sink in what you're saying.

Well I'm not entirely sure what it is that's happening lol

Of course, I wasn't laughing out loud. I don't normally type 'lol' that often. I was trying to keep it light and soften whatever was coming, even if I didn't know what that was yet.

Eighteen more minutes passed. The sense of foreboding was smothering.

Dad and I need time to digest the info and work out all the implications – so can we talk it over at the weekend?

Her tone felt serious now. My heart raced.

Okay. Well obviously whatever the story is, it doesn't change anything
Love you
Hope you're not freaking out or worried. I didn't mean to worry anyone, I just clicked on the DNA thing today and was surprised.
Love you

I felt deeply unsettled. My parents were being cagey and I couldn't tell if they had been unwittingly dropped into this obscurity, like me, or if they were hiding something.

I replied to Lucy.

Coincidence

Thanks so much for the info. I'm seeing my parents this weekend so I am going to talk to them about everything. As far as my siblings and I know, we are biologically related to our parents... they had IVF in Nottingham between 1986-1991 resulting in 2 pregnancies (my older brother in 1986 and us three, non-identical triplets, in 1991). So if you are my half sister then it is rather confusing, because it could mean my dad somehow has children he doesn't know about. Though he doesn't match the description of your donor dad...

Or it means I am not biologically related to my dad which would be quite a shock!

I have lots of questions! I'm going to sit down with my family over the weekend and see what they know :-)

In three days' time I would be heading home to celebrate Easter with the whole family. I sank into bed that night feeling a prickly sense of trepidation and a pang of adrenaline. Two tectonic plates had collided and my sense of self was shifting.

In the weeks before, I had been developing ideas for new television shows at work. Coincidentally, my strongest idea at the time was for a documentary series about the phenomenon of egg donor websites in America. It was a fascinating world that I had been researching for weeks. I had started writing a proposal to pitch to television commissioners. It read:

> 'Inconceivable' follows an egg donor agency in the US, where elite young female donors are matched with potential couples desperate to have a baby. The agency website is like Tinder for your baby's genetics.
>
> Couples can swipe left to pay $5000 – $25,000 for the donor they want. The more accomplished, intelligent, beautiful, and creative the woman, the higher the price tag.

We follow the couples desperate to get pregnant, alongside the women who decide to become egg donors. Many donors fund their university education this way, with Harvard, Yale and Stanford students being the most targeted by egg donor agencies.

But donating is not an easy ride. Donors have to go through numerous physical and psychological tests, self-administer daily injections, endure bloating, mood swings and surgery under anaesthetic. They also risk adverse long term health problems after donating such as Ovary Hyperstimulation Syndrome, haemorrhaging, or ironically, even infertility.

FACTS

- 10,000 babies are born each year to egg donors in the US
- Use of donor eggs has increased 30% since 2005
- In the UK egg donors get paid a maximum of £750 but in the US the practice is much more competitive and lucrative

Some people believe that secrets reveal themselves in small ways throughout one's life and that there is always a knowing deep within. Children pick up on glances, hesitation, avoidance. Something slightly awry. Words unspoken. For some reason, I had always been interested in the ethics of conception. As a teenager I began writing a dystopian novel about a woman whose mother was never born because she was conceived from eggs retrieved from her mother's womb while her mother was still a foetus in her grandmother's womb. It won a writing competition. In more recent years I had started a novel about restorative justice. The story followed a single woman whose son was conceived using a sperm donor then tragically killed in an accident at the age of seven. The idea of someone having a child they went through so much effort to conceive, to be taken away so suddenly was unimaginable; the kind of grief that was ripe for a complex narrative of emotional turmoil. I wanted to explore how people moved on with their lives after something so tragic happens, and how women's lives in particular are shaped by their identity as mothers.

Looking back I was probably writing about my own fears as a way to try and mitigate them. These private obsessions with conception may seem like coincidences, but perhaps they were clues.

My parents, John and Sandra, met on a blind double date in the summer of 1969, though they were not paired with each other. Seventeen-year-old Sandra – five foot two with long blonde hair and a baby face – and her friend, Lesley, wanted to watch a concert at their local rugby club but had no way of getting there or back. Small Faces and Pickettywitch were performing and everyone wanted a ticket. Lesley asked her friend Jean – a local beauty queen – to ask her boyfriend, John, to invite two friends along so that Sandra and Lesley would have an excuse to hitch a ride. Once they arrived at the gig, Sandra and Lesley made a point of disappearing into the crowd since neither were keen on John's mates, and when it was time to go home they reappeared in the car park. With his girlfriend waiting in the car, John – a lanky five foot ten, with dark hair and blue eyes – asked Sandra for a goodbye kiss on the cheek. Sandra was taken aback; how brazen of him. A few days later, he asked his ex-girlfriend for Sandra's number. John had broken up with Jean; it turned out that the beauty queen had another boyfriend in Wales.

John called Sandra at work – she was a receptionist at a caravan rental company – and she agreed to go on a date. They arranged to meet at a bus stop in Nottingham city centre, but Sandra didn't show. John decided to wait twenty minutes before accepting that he'd been stood up and headed home. Half an hour after the agreed time, Sandra arrived finally. She'd missed her bus.

Luckily, John was still standing there, having waited an extra ten minutes just in case. If he hadn't, that probably would have been the end of their love story. Their friends reckoned they wouldn't last six months because they argued so much, but fifty years later they are still together, still bickering playfully, still happy.

When they were eighteen, two of Sandra's best friends got married on the same day. One bride wore baby blue, the other baby pink. They couldn't wear white because they were both pregnant. A few months later they gave birth in beds next to each other. John and Sandra wanted a family too, but were in no rush. Ten years later, when they tried it didn't happen. They were eventually referred for fertility treatment and after four years of failed artificial insemination attempts they signed up for a new technology called IVF.

In 1986, my older brother, Tim, was born. A few years on, hoping for a sibling, they tried IVF again. But it failed. They tried again and again. Their fourth attempt was particularly demoralising. Sandra arrived at the hospital ready for an embryo transfer but was told that none of their four frozen embryos had survived the thawing process. Devastated, she was sent home empty-wombed.

By late 1990, Sandra was going through her fifth round of IVF around the same time as Mary who she'd met years before through a mutual friend. Mary had suffered with a childhood infection that had left her unable to conceive naturally. The two women quickly discovered that they shared an unlikely chain of coincidences. They had grown up on the same street and had attended the same school, a few years apart, and they had both had baby boys. Mary's son was six months younger than Tim, but the pregnancy had not been straightforward. The six-week scan showed two heartbeats and a separate empty sac. At eight weeks, Mary started feeling unwell and the midwife who administered her daily progesterone injection suspected that one of the embryos had become ectopic. Ectopic comes from the Greek *ektopos*, which means 'out of place', and accounts for approximately 2 per cent of all pregnancies, most often when the embryo becomes lodged in one of the fallopian tubes. Unfortunately these pregnancies are never viable because it is not possible to move the ectopic embryo into the womb. If the embryo is not removed – by medication or surgery – it will keep growing and risks rupturing the fallopian tube.

Mary was admitted into emergency surgery and begged the surgeon to save the other baby. Fortunately, she managed to remove the ectopic foetus and fallopian tube without disrupting the other pregnancy. Mary was told that had they waited another ten minutes she would have gone into terminal shock due to internal bleeding. Her son, Robert, was the first IVF baby to survive such a surgery and her case was published in a medical paper.

Four years later, Sandra and Mary were undergoing fertility treatment again, hoping for a sibling for their sons. To their surprise, both became pregnant with triplets. As their bellies expanded, their friendship grew and Mary and Sandra became best friends.

In May 1991, Mary gave birth to Sophie, Zoe and Matthew. Two girls and a boy. As she and her husband welcomed their three babies into the world, Sandra was lying in a room on the same wing of the hospital, sporting an impressive fifty-four-inch waist. After initially going into labour at twenty-six weeks, she had been given medication and was being kept on bed-rest for the remainder of the pregnancy. But when her friend's babies were born, she couldn't resist hobbling over to see them. Three tiny, glorious newborns.

Sixteen days after her friend gave birth, Sandra, now 31.5 weeks gestation, was having routine tests to check her kidney function. The nurse took a swab from her shin to see if urine was seeping through her skin.

'All looks okay,' the nurse said.

'What about this?' said Sandra, raising one leg to reveal the back of her thigh, heavy and turgid with fluid. The nurse gasped.

'I'll get someone to come and look.'

Soon a steady stream of medical staff were gawking at Sandra's swollen limbs and within a few hours she had been scheduled for a Caesarean section. It was a Sunday afternoon, so a team of fifteen paediatricians had to be scrambled together at short notice. Five for each premature baby.

On the evening of 2 June 1991, my parents welcomed their own triplets: Rebecca, Ruth and Joseph. Also two girls and a boy. It was like winning the lottery, Dad said. But being born is better than winning the lottery. The odds of winning the lottery are one in 45 million, whereas the odds of being born are like two million people rolling a dice at the same time and getting the same number. It's a one in 400 trillion chance. It is almost inconceivable.

Being more than two months premature, we were too small for our newborn clothes, so they dressed us in doll's clothes. We were the same size as Dad's hand, but he couldn't hold us because we were in incubators. The nurses joked that they didn't recognise Sandra as her face and body had changed so drastically since giving birth. They called her the 'incredible shrinking woman'.

While my parents marvelled at the three newest members of their family, Mary's son Matthew was struggling to survive. We were all premature and fragile, but Matthew had developed necrotising enterocolitis, an intestinal disorder that affects around 7 per cent of premature babies. It is treatable if picked up in time, but over the following days Matthew developed E. coli and then sepsis. He died two days later. He was just eighteen days old. Zoe and Sophie lost their brother before they got a chance to know him.

Despite being advised not to go while recovering from surgery, Sandra attended Matthew's funeral to support her friend.

Instead of flowers, Mary had requested that donations be sent to the neonatal unit, but Sandra ordered a basket of yellow flowers shaped like a Moses basket as well. It remains a tradition today that Mary places bright yellow flowers on his grave.

'At least you've still got the other two,' people said to Mary. Well-wishers, with good intentions no doubt. But there are no silver linings to a newborn's funeral. It is no way to comfort a bereaved parent.

We were all miracle babies – new technology had allowed us to exist – but there were supposed to be six of us. Why was one of us snatched away? While we remained triplets, overnight Zoe and Sophie became 'twins', which is how most people know them now. But to me they will always be triplets.

A few weeks later, with the five of us still in incubators on the intensive care unit, getting on with our growing, Mary was keeping watch while the other mothers had a break. She noticed my sister, Ruth, struggling to breathe. Ruth had been the smallest at birth, weighing just two pounds and fourteen ounces, and now her tiny lungs were giving up and she was turning blue. The hospital staff had been flitting around in the background, busy with their tasks, and not noticed Ruth's coughing and spluttering, her rapid deterioration. Mary ran over and raised the alarm. She saved Ruth's life.

As newborns the three of us shared everything; a pram, a bath, a cot. Breastfeeding was a rotation system: two on the breast, one on the bottle. As we got bigger, Mum and Dad invested in a triple buggy: two babies in the back, one in the front. Since I was the heaviest, I always went in the front. One day Mum picked me up first, causing Ruth and Joe to fly backwards and hit their heads on the pavement. She never did that again.

The large pram created a lot of attention. People would change direction on the street to follow Mum and talk to her. Once, a man asked if the reason she had triplets was because she'd had sex three times in one night. Dad hated the attention and they started taking us out less often.

By the time we started primary school, the Japanese craze of Tamagotchi was in full swing and for a few weeks we carried around our pocket-sized digital pets – until the headteacher confiscated them because they were becoming too disruptive in lessons. Desperate to keep them alive, Mum took the Tamagotchis with her to college, where she was doing a diploma in computing at the time. Her tutor and the other students thought it was hilarious watching her trying to concentrate in class while juggling three Tamagotchis at once. Mum is a great multi-tasker. She had to be.

Growing up, Zoe, Sophie, Ruth and I were inseparable. We still call each other 'wombies' because we've been friends since the womb. Despite going to different schools, we spent the holidays together, exploring adventure playgrounds and waterparks. Our mums didn't want my brother Joe to feel left out, being the only boy among four girls the same age, so he was always allowed to invite a friend to our group play dates. As it happened both of Joe's best friends growing up were called Matthew. So there was always a Matthew by our side. He was always with us.

Unlike us, Zoe and Sophie were told from a young age that they had been conceived by IVF. In fact, they knew we had been too and were told to keep it a secret from us, which they did. When eleven-year-old Zoe and Sophie joined a Catholic high school, their new friends were interested in the fact that they were twins. Zoe and Sophie proudly proclaimed that they had been conceived with IVF, but the children started talking, and then the teachers did too. It cannot be a coincidence that during their next RE lesson, their teacher began by quoting the Bible:

> For you formed my inward parts;
> you knitted me together in my mother's womb.
> - Psalm 139:13, English Standard Version

She told the story of Hannah and how 'the Lord had closed her womb'.

'If God intended a woman to be pregnant he would grant her this naturally, therefore any child born through IVF will forever be a sin,' the teacher admonished the class.

Flooded with frustration, Sophie stood up and walked out of the classroom. She was given a detention.

Any child born through IVF will forever be a sin. Not our parents, not the doctors. Us. I hope with all my soul that no children are made to feel so ashamed and unworthy today. No matter how we arrived into this world, we all deserve to be here.

Sophie is still one of my best friends. She has wavy blonde hair, a dazzling smile and the word GROOVY tattooed on her thigh. We regularly have deep conversations about our lives and we also quote *Mean Girls* to each other constantly. We both studied at universities in London and have been there for each other; always available for a hug, a cup of tea and some therapeutic pottery painting. When I introduce friends to Sophie and they ask how we know each other, it's hard to put into words. She's like a sister. We met in the womb, we say. We've been friends since the day we were born.

When we talk about the Catholic school incident these days we both agree that if naturally conceived babies are a gift from God, then who's to say the work of the scientists that made us wasn't a gift too? In any case, we're probably lost causes. Catholicism deems sex before marriage, masturbation and homosexuality to be sinful too. Sophie is married to a woman, and if she has children one day she may require fertility treatment.

But for all of her supposed sins, Sophie is the most generous, kind and caring person I know. People say that all the time, though with her it really is true. She is a paediatric intensive care nurse and has dedicated her life to looking after the most critically ill newborns, while training up the next generation of nurses to do the same. In her spare time she stitches handmade quilts for babies. Over the years Sophie has helped save the lives of hundreds of tiny babies like Ruth and Matthew.

Shame

Definition

1. A painful feeling caused by wrong or foolish behaviour
2. A regrettable or unfortunate situation
3. Loss of honour or respect

Three days after I was matched with a 'half-sister' on the DNA website, I boarded a train to my parents' house in Nottinghamshire. Mum picked me up from the station and after some brief updates and mundane chat about the journey, I couldn't wait any longer.

'So are we going to talk about it?'

'I'm not going to discuss it now,' she replied, curtly.

I leaned back in my seat and gazed ahead at the moonlit country roads. It was late when we arrived home so I went straight to bed, feeling disturbed by her abruptness; fearing what was coming.

I didn't sleep well and in the early morning I tiptoed out of bed and headed for the kitchen. While my siblings and their partners slept, I made cups of tea and coaxed Mum and Dad into the living room. They shuffled in at a distance behind me, reluctantly, like giant magnets I was repelling. Mum closed the door behind us and locked it. We sat down in silence, Mum on the sofa next to me and Dad in his armchair, all facing towards the black television screen. Dread stirred in my gut.

'Can you just tell me what's going on?' I asked.

Dad perched his elbow on the armrest, hiding his face from my view with his hand. Mum sighed into the thickening air.

'When we went for fertility treatment for my blocked fallopian tubes,' she began, 'they also discovered that Dad's sperm wasn't viable.'

She stared blankly ahead. I could tell how hard it was for her to say these words aloud.

'It was a double whammy of bad news,' she continued. 'And so the clinic offered us a sperm donor.'

My heart sank. I had my answer, finally. The tiny bubble of hope I'd been naively protecting was punctured.

'No one else has ever known. It was just me, Dad and the hospital staff,' Mum said, 'and they encouraged us not to tell anyone.'

I fixated on the ornaments above the fireplace – two golden brass dogs, one on either side – stoutly perched there since before we were born. I didn't know what to say, so I just nodded. It was a relief to be sitting in the truth, dank and disappointing though it was.

Mum motioned her eyes over to Dad who was sobbing underneath his cloistered hand. It was a look she'd given me before. Give him some attention, it conveyed, he won't ask for it himself. I stood up and moved towards him, arching my body over his convulsing frame. I'd only seen him cry like this once before in my life, when his mum had died twenty years earlier.

'It's okay, Dad,' I muffled into his shoulder, gripping his arm.

He placed his hand on top of mine but said nothing. I held him a few moments longer, then sat back down on the sofa next to Mum.

I was appalled that my stupid curiosity had done this. I wanted to take back the DNA results, forget it all happened and go back to before. I wanted Dad to stop being upset.

'I'm sorry,' I said, my belly knotting around this unfamiliar territory. 'It doesn't change anything.'

Dad was still bent over and shaking. Mum still stared vacantly ahead. I had trodden on a land mine that I didn't know was there.

'So, did you pick him out of a catalogue or something?' I asked, not able to bear the silence.

'We just let the hospital choose,' Mum replied.

'Oh.' It surprised me that they had left such a big decision to strangers. 'But I've always been told I look like Dad,' I said, as if that might make it true again. 'So they obviously did a good job of choosing.'

More silence.

'Lucy, the half-sister, messaged me and said apparently he was a young medical student, six foot with green eyes.'

Neither of them said anything.

'We never thought you'd find out,' Mum said. 'How were we to know that DNA websites would exist one day?'

I nodded slowly. It was fair enough, who could have predicted that?

'We'll have to tell everyone now,' Dad murmured eventually.

'No, wait,' I interjected, then paused. I looked at the floor. 'I don't know if we should.'

Dad lifted his head.

'I wish I hadn't found out,' I said, hoping it would comfort him, though I still meant it. 'We don't need to tell them.'

The thought of breaking three more hearts that day was too much to bear. We couldn't do an Easter egg hunt if we were all crying. I had the whole day planned out. I didn't want to ruin the weekend for everyone.

'I've kept it a secret so far, I can just keep it,' I offered.

'That's a lot to keep on your own, darling,' said Mum.

'I know but I'm used to it. I basically do it for my job. It's fine.'

A few moments passed. I had so many questions but didn't know how to ask them without upsetting Dad even more. I was still my mother's biological daughter; they had fixed her fertility problem but not his. An invisible line had been drawn between us, and I hated it.

'So we won't tell them, then?' Dad confirmed.

I nodded.

'Okay,' he said and stood up. 'Sandra, add champagne to the shopping list and let's crack on with Easter.'

He unlocked the door and walked out. Back into the world where he was our dad and there was no more to it. I wished I could have followed him back into that world.

I am not sure if I had meant that I didn't want to tell everyone else that day, that month or that year. I'm not sure if I meant forever. I did not know what people were supposed to do in these situations; what the 'right' thing to do was. All I wanted was to undo all the sadness.

Mum and I were left alone, sitting on the sofa. It felt like the energy had been sucked out of the room. From our whole lives. What a mess I had caused.

'Be careful who else you talk to about it,' she warned. 'Some people don't understand these things.'

I sensed some shame between her words, some residue of the past crystallising as she spoke. It was to remain a secret in this family, I understood, but beyond that, what were the rules? Be careful, yes, but not 'don't tell anyone'. There was some wiggle room, which I felt strangely grateful for. Guilty too.

Mum invited me outside to look at the new trees and shrubs she'd planted. We walked around the area of the garden where my grandma's ashes are buried, Dad's mum, underneath a delicate bush with red leaves.

'Dad wanted to tell you when you were teenagers,' Mum said. My mind, swirling, stopped for a second. 'But I persuaded him not to.'

'Why?'

'Because I didn't think he was doing it for the right reasons,' she said. 'He wanted to know if you all loved him for him or just because he was your dad.'

A lump formed in my throat. I had not known a side to my dad like this, a side that seemed so fragile and insecure about his place in our lives. My dad, a joiner who has spent his life on top of church roofs in the snapping cold of winter, never complaining, and in the blistering heat of summer, never wearing suncream. A woodworker for more than fifty years; a master of his craft. A man whose hands are thick and coarse like sandpaper. Always creating things for us from pieces of leftover wood: bookcases, picture frames, a dollhouse. Extensions of his heart and sometimes extensions of our house: a bathroom, a conservatory, a cabin in the woods. Labours of his love. He had built our home, he was our home.

I pictured us all as teenagers, reacting to the news that he wasn't our biological father. I was an exasperating teenager, known to shout back and slam doors, but I knew I would not have done so for this. The idea that my dad questioned whether or why we loved him was unbearable. The reason children love their parents is ineffable, because they are everything. For those of us lucky enough to have parents like mine, they are the precious kind of everything. Our parents are history and meaning and the roots that anchor us deep into the earth. They are the earth, the soil.

Mum and I drifted around the saplings in silence.

'What do our birth certificates say?' I asked.

'In the early days they used a technique where they would mix some of the father's sperm with the donor sperm, so they could say there was a chance. But I don't think they did that with you. For the birth certificate they said you can put down your husband's name or "unknown". So it says Dad's name.'

We wandered around the tulip garden, admiring all the different colours we'd chosen from bulb packets. White, red-fringed with yellow, dark purple. They had bloomed and were top-heavy now, bending in all directions.

For my family, Easter has historically been less about Jesus and more about gin. For years we've used the long weekend as an annual excuse to round up the family troops, drink cocktails and play silly games. That Saturday continued as planned; eggs were hidden, paper riddles were strategically placed and everyone donned their bunny masks for the big egg hunt, competing in pairs. I hosted an Easter-themed quiz and we drank 'champagne' from Aldi. We laughed and we bickered and everything on the outside looked the same.

As evening descended, we moved into the kitchen and carried on drinking and chatting, while Mum made dinner. On my way to the bathroom I passed through the hallway, when I heard a little voice call my name.

'Becka.'

I turned around and peered into the darkness.

'Becka?'

I could make out the shape of my dad sitting in his armchair in the living room, lights off, in the dark.

'Becka, come over here,' he whispered.

While most people call me Rebecca or Bex these days, Becka is the name my dad has called me since I was a child. I scuttled in and perched myself between the armchair and the radiator, below the windowsill, something I had often done as a child to keep warm. The two of us had spent hundreds of evenings watching reruns of *All Creatures Great and Small* and *Only Fools and Horses* like this, side by side.

'It doesn't change anything, does it?' Dad asked.

'No, of course not,' I replied. 'It just shows how much you wanted us.'

We sat for a few moments like that; an island of stillness, distant voices humming in the background.

'If anything it makes me appreciate you even more,' I said.

Dad smiled, his eyes glinting from the lights that reached us from the kitchen, where everyone else was.

When people uncover difficult secrets, they often say it's not the truth that hurts the most, it's the lying. But lying is a strong word, pregnant with emotion and enmity. I was not angry at my parents; I did not blame them for concealing the truth. When secrets are buried so deep for so long, it's not uncommon for the gatekeepers to believe the stories themselves. In any case, no doubt they thought they were protecting us. Agreements had been made in full faith, in collusion with medical professionals and sealed shut with the wax stamp of stigma. No one else needed to know. But now the seal had been broken.

Despite understanding, rationally, the reasons for the secret, I felt blindsided. It was like stepping into the road a second too early, or dropping a precious ring down the drain. Catastrophic but so quick. Something that nearly didn't happen but changes everything. And it was my fault. Contending with my parents' emotions, I felt like there was no room for my own.

While guilt arises from acts of wrongdoing, shame is 'not a separate act, but a revelation of the whole self,' wrote the American sociologist Helen Merrell Lynd in her 1958 book *On Shame and the Search for Identity*. 'The thing that has been exposed is what I am.'

Where guilt is feeling bad about something we have *done*, shame is feeling bad about who we *are*. Guilt is often short-lived, while shame is durable and affects us on a more fundamental level. According to Lynd, 'Guilt can be expiated', but shame 'is retained'. Guilt comes after a conscious action, whereas 'the shameful situation frequently takes one by surprise'. It is the abruptness, the unforeseen nature of the news that begets shame, regardless of how large or small the actual revelation is. Lynd describes it as being 'caught off guard, or off base, caught unawares, made a fool of', which is precisely how I felt.

We cannot protect ourselves from what we do not see coming. We are forced to question what we thought we knew. 'We have acted on the assumption of being one kind of person living in one kind of surroundings,' Lynd writes, 'and unexpectedly, violently, we discover that these assumptions are false.' The secret felt like an intrusion, an invasion of my whole self. How could it not? I felt embarrassed that I no longer knew where I came from, and neither did my parents. The message was clear: our story was shameful, unpalatable to society, so it needed to be kept a secret. My immediate response was to stop the shame from spreading, as though it were a contagious disease.

I would not tell my siblings.

Curious

Definition

1. A desire to know or learn something
2. Strange, unusual

I continued messaging my half-sister, Lucy, and she told me she had a twin sister, Libby, who also worked in London. I let her know what had happened at the weekend.

I spoke to my parents and they told me that we were conceived by a sperm donor. Which was a shock . . . and something I had never considered my whole life.

It wasn't the news I was hoping for of course, I love my dad, and it raises all kinds of questions, but I understand why they didn't tell us and don't blame them at all. They didn't think we would ever find out, but I guess no one predicted this advancement in technology would happen so soon and make it so easy for people to know more about their genetics!

We shed a few tears, but we also had a lovely weekend together and it's made me appreciate them more than ever. My dad is still my amazing dad and I couldn't ask for a better family. They were planning to tell my siblings too after they talked to me, but I suggested we don't, or at least not for a while, until I've had longer to process it. I'm not sure what benefit there is to them finding out.

I asked if Lucy and her sister were around to meet up for a coffee the following week. Since I couldn't talk to my own siblings, they were the next best thing.

The following Sunday the three of us met for a roast dinner at a pub in east London. I was nervous walking in, but Lucy and Libby were friendly, funny and easy to talk to. We noticed we all had the same colour hair and were about the same height, Lucy just slightly taller. I was amazed to discover that Libby lived in Dalston, just down the road from my flat. We were born in Nottingham but had somehow ended up living less than two miles apart.

'So how did you both find out?' I asked.

'Oh, well, that's a funny story—' Lucy laughed.

'Our parents got divorced when we were eleven,' Libby interjected, 'and our mum asked us who we wanted to live with: her or our dad. And then she said, he's not your real dad.'

'Oh my god,' I said. 'That's a terrible way to find out.'

'I know. It was pretty traumatic,' Libby replied, smiling.

'You'll notice we have a pretty dark sense of humour,' Lucy said.

'That makes three of us,' I said.

Discovering such a big secret by accident in your late twenties is shocking, but having it used as ammunition for custody during your parents' divorce must have been brutal. They seemed blasé about it now, but it must have been heartbreaking. At least they had each other, I thought. In lieu of my own siblings, I was grateful to have them to talk to.

We took photographs, trying to decipher any genetic resemblance, and drank cocktails into the evening. When the time came to pay the bill, each of us put down the same debit card and I took a picture of our three purple cards lined up together in the little dish.

Before the secret emerged, I'd had a challenging few days at work. *The Family Secret* documentary I was working on followed the story of a woman who had been sexually abused as a child by her brother. We had interviewed the family and were filming them through a formal process of restorative justice. When I got home after a particularly heavy day of filming, I felt like I needed to vent to Sam. I was outraged by the after-effects of such abuse and couldn't make sense of some of the things I'd heard that day. Sam listened and asked questions, but he didn't understand the nuances of child abuse and I felt like he was inadvertently blaming the victim. I tried to explain, but he didn't get it and the whole conversation made me feel worse.

'Stop worrying,' Sam said. 'It's not your problem. You need to stop taking on other people's burdens.'

'But it's my job,' I replied, frustrated. 'It's not helpful to tell me to just stop worrying. I need to get it off my chest. These are real people, and this stuff is so much more common than people think.'

'Well,' Sam huffed, 'it sounds like you don't want my advice. It sounds like you just want someone to listen to you.'

'Yes,' I said, deflated. 'That's exactly what I want.'

As my partner, Sam thought it was his job to come up with solutions, but really I just wanted someone to listen and agree that, yes, the world was confusing and terrible sometimes and some things can't be fixed. Sam found it depressing to talk about these kinds of issues and I couldn't blame him. He had not signed up for a career dealing with the upsetting intricacies of sexual assault and incompetent justice systems. In a way, I envied him. I wished I didn't care so much, I wished I didn't know so much.

After Sam had gone to bed, I found a therapist online and arranged an appointment. I would have to pay a stranger to listen to me instead. It was disappointing but necessary. Two days later, I walked into an attic room, above a pizza restaurant a few streets away. The therapist was a boyish, blonde woman in her thirties who specialised in 'existential therapy'. During our first session we discussed the reasons for me being there: primarily to talk about my job and my relationship, I said. After fifty minutes, I tapped her portable contactless machine with my card and walked back into the world, feeling exposed but a little lighter.

By the time the following week's session rolled around, I had found out about the sperm donor secret. When I told her, the therapist looked shocked; neither of us had been expecting such a revelation in real time. From then on it became the main event of our sessions, pushing everything else into the corner. Unpacking my feelings over the next few months, I realised that it wasn't the secret, or even the shock of finding out that had most upset me, it was having to accept that my dad was not mine in the same way any more. There was a kind of grief in realising that we were not biologically related and I was mourning my connection to him. I cried when I realised this out loud and the therapist passed me a box of tissues. The role my dad played in my life had not changed, but the integrity of our relationship – as genetic father and daughter – had been broken, and I hated it because I loved him. I wanted our similarities to be backed up with blood; inherited and authentic. Our shared idiosyncrasies; our love of gin and tonic, long baths, the Brontë sisters, Christmas and the comedy genius of Caroline Aherne.

'How do you feel about the secret being kept from you?' the therapist asked.

'Well,' I said, 'sometimes it helps me to think about the earth spinning, and how our planet is just one tiny dot in the universe. And how in ten thousand years' time none of this will matter or mean anything.'

'Hmm,' she murmured. 'It's interesting. I asked you a question about your feelings and you gave me an answer about the universe.'

'Um, okay.'

'You tend to zoom out,' she said. 'About as far away from your feelings as you can get.'

'Oh. I had no idea I was doing that.'

My tendency to hurtle through space was probably an unconscious way of avoiding my emotions, we agreed. Looking at things from a vast perspective – through a super-wide lens – gets you off the hook for dealing with anything more intimately. It was a coping technique.

At the time, I was directing my first documentary for broadcast television, camera-assisting another and developing several others, all of them challenging subjects. But I was at the stage in my career when I needed to prove myself, particularly as a female director, for whom opportunities to direct and self-shoot felt sparse. I did not need any more things to worry about, the people I was filming had enough problems of their own. My siblings didn't need to know the truth and neither did I. I wanted to forgive my parents, jump on a space rocket and fly away.

When I read Helen Merrell Lynd's book on shame, five years after that therapy session, it was the first time I truly started to make sense of what was going on. 'Experience of shame,' she writes, 'may call into question, not only one's own adequacy and the validity of the codes of one's immediate society, but the meaning of the universe itself.' Her words are a language for what I could not express at the time. 'The paradox,' she explains, is that while shame is 'an isolating, highly personal experience', it is also 'peculiarly related to one's conception of the universe, and of one's place in it'.

The discovery had not just got me questioning my own family

and the medical ecosystem surrounding sperm donation but the whole world and the entire universe. I found myself panicking about what else might be hidden from me. What else did I not know?

I often woke up in the middle of the night like I'd been electrocuted. It was as if my brain had been bickering with itself and needed an answer urgently. My subconscious seemed to ask the same questions over and over. Who am I? Who is the sperm donor? Will I ever find out? Do I already know him? Have I passed him in the street?

Every man between the age of fifty and seventy became a suspect. I worked with loads of men that age, could one of them be him? I would probably never know.

One day, while at work, I messaged Sam:

I just had a moment where I felt like I was gonna faint or be sick ... like an out of body experience where you feel like your entire life has been a lie or you are living in an alternate universe ... I'm not sure I've processed the whole sperm donor thing properly yet.

He reassured me, but there was no handbook for this kind of situation. I felt pretty alone. A few weeks later, I went to a work party, held in my boss's garden. It was the first time I'd seen the colleague I'd had a conversation with after logging on to the DNA website on the day it happened. We sat next to each other around the garden table, sipping beers.

'What happened with the DNA website stuff?' she asked.

'Oh ...' I paused. 'It wasn't very good news in the end.' I hoped my vagueness might end the conversation.

'Oh, I'm sorry,' she replied. 'What did you find out?'

I hesitated. 'Erm, well, I found out I was conceived with a sperm donor.'

'Oh my gosh, and you didn't know? That must have been a shock.'

Our other colleagues fell quiet and started listening in. Everyone wanted to know the full story and asked me questions in quick succession. They were investigative filmmakers, after all. I answered them, but it felt knotty and wrong saying the words out loud, and too intimate for a group situation, especially in front of junior colleagues I didn't know very well.

When I left the party, I walked to the tube station with a young colleague who had been working with us for a few months. She was asking more questions and I told her how strange it felt to talk to colleagues about it all when my own siblings didn't know.

'Oh my god, your siblings don't know?' she raised her voice. 'That's insane. You *have* to tell them. They have a right to know!'

'But what if it makes things worse?' I said. 'My brother is struggling with his mental health at the moment. My dad has a heart issue and my big brother is about to get married. What if they react badly and something happens? It doesn't feel like the right time.' I believed what I was saying, but I could also hear myself; it sounded like I was making excuses. 'Do they really *need* to know?'

When she got off at her stop I felt irritated and defensive, like I had been told off unfairly. She didn't know me or anything about my family. She hadn't been thrown headfirst into this absurd situation. I wanted sympathy for being put in such an awkward position, but I felt cornered and blamed. I was very careful about who else I told after that.

Shame is 'isolating, alienating, incommunicable,' writes Lynd. 'Experiences of shame appear to embody the root meaning of the word – to uncover, to expose, to wound. They are experiences of exposure, exposure of peculiarly sensitive, intimate, vulnerable aspects of the self.'

What could be more vulnerable and intimate than your own conception, the circumstances of your own existence?

When I arrived home that evening I received a text from my boss, a man in his mid-fifties and one of the most accomplished executive producers in the television industry. He had been developing a programme about 'DNA Detectives' for a broadcaster and hoped I might cast my eye over the proposal. He suggested I add in my own story as an anonymous case study since I now had 'lived experience'.

I sighed – it was more work on top of my already intense workload – but I agreed. I understood why he had asked me, and was flattered that he thought I could add something valuable, yet it felt insensitive to ask so incredibly soon. He was on a deadline for the channel, he said, and needed it done the next day. I stayed up late editing the document and sent it back, feeling empty.

Two years later, I would see him at a TV awards party, a few months after the birth of his first child. He looked better than I'd ever seen him, with a wide grin and sparkly eyes. I was surprised he had become a father at his age, but I was happy for him. He seemed totally besotted with his son.

At one point in the evening he came over and asked how I'd been getting on since the news about my family.

'Okay thanks. My siblings still don't know, but I think it's for the best.'

He leaned over. 'I've not really told anyone this,' he whispered, 'but we actually used a sperm donor too.'

For better or worse, my parents have brought up four children who are curious about the world. Everyone, aside from me, has forged a career in the sciences – completing degrees in physics, engineering and zoology – asking questions about the world, how it functions and what we can do to improve it.

My sister, Ruth, is incredibly passionate about animals, particularly marine life. She has been a guest speaker at the Natural History Museum in London and visited every continent in the world, most recently sailing to Antarctica as a research scientist for a whale conservation project.

An engineering and neuroscience graduate, our brother Joe is quirky, detail-oriented and constantly interrogating why things are the way they are. He works as a support technician for the University of Nottingham, plays fastpitch softball for Great Britain and can always be relied upon for advice about health and fitness.

As a journalist and filmmaker, my career has involved asking deep questions about society, sociology and culture. When I uncovered the secret, I was presented with the scientific facts, but I wanted to know more about how it happened and what it meant. I wanted to understand how good parents like mine could lie to their children about something so important for three decades. I wanted to speak to the people involved in the 'making' of me and my siblings and examine infertility in the context of history, politics and religion. How do science and love collide? What issues are we still wrestling with? How did we get here?

The journalist inside me was eager to learn more and get closer to the truth. I wanted to gather the evidence, interview the witnesses and cross-examine my own conception.

Baby

Definition

1. A very young child
2. A lover or spouse
3. Be overprotective towards

On 18 May 1971, the front cover of American magazine *Look* featured a photograph of a seven-week-old human embryo in the palm of a hand. The picture had been taken by a man called Landrum Shettles, holding the camera in one hand and the embryo – curled up in its amniotic sac – in the other. Above the photo, in large white print, the headline stated:

TAKING LIFE IN OUR OWN HANDS
A historic step: The test-tube baby is coming

John Coxon and Sandra Lemon were not aware of this magazine cover, nor could they have known how the technology, bubbling in the background, might affect them one day. In 1971 very few people had heard of a 'test-tube baby'.

Instead, twenty-year-old John and Sandra were planning their wedding day; a simple affair with forty people and reception at a local pub. Sandra had bought a second-hand wedding dress from the ad mag for £2. She was earning £12 a week as an office temp in a coal-fuelled power station, so it was a bargain. The dress was floor-length broderie anglaise with long sleeves, tapered in slightly below the bust. She wore pearls around her neck, a puffy netted veil and held a miniature bouquet of pink orchids, wrapped in white ribbon. Her hair was pinned up, with a middle parting and a couple of loose ringlets framing her face. John wore an oversized grey suit, pink tie with matching handkerchief and fashionable mid-length sideburns. They were married at the local village church. At the reception they smiled as they cut into their three-tier fruit cake. It was tradition to serve the bottom two layers at the wedding and save the top layer for their first child's christening. They saved the cake, but two years later when they moved house, they would open the box to find the white icing had turned yellow. The cake was mouldy.

The day after the ceremony, the newlyweds set off for their honeymoon in Salcombe, Devon. To afford it, they'd had to sell John's car, a pale blue Mini with orange stripes, so they made the five-hour journey south in Sandra's car, also a Mini – dark blue, no stripes. But during the drive they experienced a serious oil leak. John spent the first two days of the honeymoon out on the road, under the car, trying to fix it. The bedsheets at the B&B were made of blue silk, which looked lovely but was impractical. Throughout the night they kept slipping off the bed.

The man holding the embryo on the magazine cover that year, Landrum Shettles, was described as awkward and eccentric by some, and a genius by others. He tended to rely on his own memory rather than recording clinical notes, and while other medical professionals published their research in scientific journals, Shettles often went straight to the tabloid press. In 1971, he published a book called *How to Choose the Sex of Your Baby* in which readers could follow the 'Shettles Method' to influence the sex of their child by douching the vagina with vinegar and altering the timing or position of their intercourse. The public lapped it up, and the book sold more than a million copies. But while Shettles claimed a 75 per cent success rate for his methods, his fellow scientists were sceptical. His hospital superiors resented the media attention and were embarrassed by his links to the hospital where they worked.

Attempting to clip his influence on real patients, Shettles' bosses reduced his duties and deprived him of any patient care or research roles. And yet he was always wandering around the hospital corridors. At all hours of day or night, he floated around in his white coat like a ghost. Some colleagues wanted rid of him while others took pity since he had a wife and seven children, who rarely saw him thanks to his preference for sleeping in a hospital cubby-hole instead of at home. Each night he would pull out a bed in his makeshift office, surrounded by stacks of medical papers and his odd collection of clocks, all ticking to slightly different times.

By 1972, across the Atlantic Ocean, the front cover of British glossy magazine *Nova* was featuring a smiling baby in a white fleece nappy. On its belly was stamped 'Department of Reproduction' and next to it the headline:

THE PERFECT BABY OR THE BIGGEST THREAT SINCE THE ATOM BOMB?

The concept of test-tube babies was starting to enter the public consciousness, but so far scientists had only achieved fertilisation outside the womb; no one anywhere in the world had brought about a pregnancy or birth.

Meanwhile, Sandra was celebrating her twenty-first birthday. John had bought her twenty-one red roses and they were making plans to go cherry-picking in rural France for a season. Then they saw an advert on television for 'ten pound poms' and changed their minds. Many of their friends were settling down – married with mortgages and more mouths to feed – but Sandra and John saw that kind of life as a millstone around their necks. They wanted to travel, explore the world and enjoy their youth. The ten pound pom scheme sounded perfect.

In what was one of the largest planned migrations of the twentieth century, the campaign encouraged young couples to emigrate to Australia – requiring only the £10 administration fee – on the condition that they stayed for at least two years. The British and Australian governments sought young, white, British couples to go forth and multiply as part of their new 'Populate or Perish' policy. John and Sandra drove down to London for an interview, pretending they wanted to move to Australia for the foreseeable future rather than to use the scheme as a subsidised opportunity to go on an adventure. They wished to emigrate to Australia forever, they told the officials, and raise a family there.

In April 1973, they boarded the SS *Australis*, a 2,250-capacity ocean liner and former US Navy ship, in Southampton. With the Suez Canal closed they had to go the long way round. There is a photograph of Sandra sitting in their tiny, basic cabin room, propped up against two single bunk beds. She is perched next to a fruit bowl, wearing a paisley pink-and-white mini-dress, and looks deeply unimpressed. It would be a long six weeks.

When the ship docked in Cape Town, South Africa, John asked someone to take a photo of them in front of Table Mountain, and they posted it back home to his mum, Louie. In the picture Sandra is wearing a floaty pink top and when Louie saw it she was convinced her daughter-in-law was pregnant. Later, when the couple returned to England after two and a half years, Louie would accuse them of having a baby and leaving it in Australia. Sandra was more bemused than appalled. She was in her early twenties and completely disinterested in babies. Louie was always trying to get her to hold other people's children.

'I'll just wait to hold my own,' Sandra would reply.

Perhaps haunted by her own stillbirth, Louie worried she would never become a grandma.

Eventually John and Sandra arrived in Perth, Western Australia. As they were beginning their new lives on the other side of the world, eleven thousand miles away a couple from Florida were walking into their doctor's office in New York.

Dr William Sweeney, an infertility specialist, had been seeing Doris and John Del Zio for a number of years and was running out of options to help them have a baby. Twenty-nine-year-old Doris had already undergone three surgeries to clear her blocked fallopian tubes, followed by months of artificial insemination, resulting in a single miscarriage.

'They can put a man on the moon,' Doris said, 'isn't there some way scientists can figure out how to help me have a child?'

Sweeney admitted that there was one more thing they could try but it was experimental and had only ever been successful in mice and rabbits. It was called in vitro fertilisation. *In vitro* being Latin for 'in glass'. Scientists around the world were trying to master the procedure – extracting eggs from a woman's ovaries and placing them in a glass container with her partner's sperm to create an embryo – but so far none had succeeded. Sweeney contacted Landrum Shettles, who had been doing research on egg physiology and fertilisation since the 1940s, and asked for his help. The Del Zios enthusiastically agreed to whatever it was they were signing up for and completed some makeshift paperwork.

On 12 September 1973, Sweeney made an incision in Doris's abdomen and extracted some follicular fluid from her ovaries, hoping it would contain at least one egg. He placed the fluid inside two corked test tubes, shrouded them in bubble wrap and handed them to John Del Zio. John was instructed to take them a hundred blocks north to Columbia-Presbyterian Hospital, where Shettles was waiting. John put the eggs in his jacket pocket, holding the tubes close to his chest to keep them warm, and hailed a cab. When he arrived fifteen minutes later, Shettles asked John to produce a semen sample. The doctor then poured the semen into one of the test tubes before placing the mixture in an incubator.

What happened next would become the subject of a highly publicised court case and a book by Robin Marantz Henig called *Pandora's Baby*. It would set a precedent regarding IVF treatment in the United States for decades to come. But on that day in September 1973, it was less like Pandora's baby and more like Schrödinger's embryo.

In passing, Shettles had told a colleague about his plan to implant an embryo into his patient. That colleague told another who got in touch with the hospital's chief of obstetrics and gynecology, Raymond Vande Wiele, a Belgian doctor, raised in the Catholic Church and highly regarded around the world in his field. Vande Wiele summoned Shettles to his office and Shettles arrived to find his test tube on the table in front of him, uncorked, at room temperature. Next to it was a tape recorder already running.

Shettles was reprimanded for not getting clearance for the 'experiment' from Columbia's human experimentation committee. In not doing so, Vande Wiele said, he was putting all of the hospital's future funding at risk. Vande Wiele then read out loud from an article in the *New England Journal of Medicine* about how cautiously a pair of British scientists called Patrick Steptoe and Robert Edwards were proceeding with this new IVF technology; not implanting embryos until they could rule out the likelihood of defects.

'I mean, here on one side,' said Vande Wiele, 'the English investigators are concerned about ethical problems and Dr Shettles is not.' What kind of a position, he asked, did it put not only their department but the entire medical school in?

Shettles said that because the procedure involved a patient of Sweeney's and the implantation was to be performed at New York Hospital, he did not think Columbia's approval was required. After a lengthy and heated conversation, Vande Wiele said he would dispose of the test tube. On the way out Shettles offered to throw it away too. It is not clear if anyone ever checked to see if fertilisation had actually taken place, but whatever happened to the test tube, we can be sure that no baby came from it.

Shettles called Doris that evening and apologised profusely, telling her the procedure had been cancelled because a senior colleague disagreed with it. She was distraught. She kept asking why a man she didn't know would take away her chance to have a baby. In the months that followed she became depressed, anxious and socially withdrawn. A few days before Christmas 1973, on their fifth wedding anniversary, she wrote a letter to her husband apologising for failing to give him the child he wanted.

'I'm in a vacuum now,' Doris wrote. 'Too much has happened to me in the last few months, somehow I have to bring myself back to normal, I don't know how. So far, you haven't been able to help me, I don't know who can help, but I have to find help somewhere. It scares me. I don't like being in this vacuum.' She signs off the letter, 'Sorry this anniversary isn't a happy one for you, it's all my fault and I can't help it.'

In the new year Doris returned to the operating theatre to have a fibroid removed from her uterus, but was told there was little else they could do to help with her infertility. She was so heartbroken and humiliated, she said, that she stopped wanting to look at her husband, never mind have sex with him. The last time they had made love was on his fifty-sixth birthday, the day before she was admitted into hospital for the IVF procedure.

A few months later, Doris collapsed in a department store, waking to find a retail assistant hovering over her, asking if she was okay. When Doris looked down she saw that her arms were filled with baby clothes. It was June, nine months since the procedure. Her subconscious mind had given birth to a baby.

Not long afterwards, the Del Zios filed a lawsuit against Dr

Vande Wiele, Columbia University and Presbyterian Hospital for 'intentional infliction of emotional distress', seeking compensation of $1.5 million.

In the north of England, gynaecologist Patrick Steptoe was seeing his own patients who were suffering from infertility. They often left his office feeling disappointed, he wrote in his memoir *A Matter of Life*, but there was one word in particular he hated using. *Never.*

'The verdict of "never", even when softly-spoken, leaves the woman shaking, empty, her face too naked, her private grief too unconcealed.'

For all of human history there have been people who could not conceive children, and for many of them there was simply nothing that could be done. Steptoe wanted to change that, thanks in part to his mother, Grace, who had influenced his route into gynaecology. She was 'very conscious of the rights of women and the wrongs done to them' and had 'always gently suggested that one day I might be able to help them'.

After working in London hospitals and learning about the 'mystery' of infertility, Steptoe realised it 'was a complaint of two people, not of one' – as was so often presumed – and saw first-hand the lifelong unhappiness it could cause. To some, he wrote, it even became an obsession.

> Sometimes it disrupted what otherwise might have been an amiable marriage. There were men who, fearful that they were sterile, became impotent. There were women who, desperate, tried folk remedies, prayed for long hours in a darkened room, or visited special shrines.

After being turned down for highly competitive consultant jobs in London, Steptoe established a practice in Oldham, Greater

Manchester, becoming an expert in surgery using a laparoscope, a thin tube with an optical-fibre light that is inserted into the abdomen for medical procedures such as the diagnosis and treatment of blocked fallopian tubes. Sometimes this improved the couples' chances of conceiving, but often it didn't.

Two hundred and fifty miles away, at the University of Cambridge, a physiologist called Robert Edwards was studying genetic abnormalities in mice embryos, with the goal of eventually moving on to humans. By the late 1960s, Edwards and his colleague, Barry Bavister, had managed to fertilise sperm and egg outside the body, in a Petri dish, an extraordinary breakthrough. But to obtain eggs, Edwards had to wait for strips of ovarian tissue to become available from women undergoing gynaecological surgery in the hands of his friend, Molly Rose, a gynaecologist who delivered one of his daughters. Rose was based in London and the phone calls to come and collect the tissue could be sporadic and often very last-minute. The process was also highly unethical since the women were not made aware that their eggs were being taken away and experimented on. Edwards needed to find a better way to remove eggs, so when he came across an article in a medical journal about laparoscopy written by a gynaecologist called Steptoe, he approached him and asked for help.

Along with Edwards' assistant, Jean Purdy, the group forged ahead with their research, trying to create life outside the womb. The way Edwards and Steptoe wrote about these early days, it is hard not to be moved by the magic of it.

> A beautiful disc of fetal cells, the beginning of the fetus as it started its journey towards life. Light, transparent, floating, expanding slightly, but still smaller than a pinpoint: there they were, four excellent blastocysts. The intrinsic beauty of it!

In 1971 they applied for funding from the British Medical Research Council to continue their experiments, but the council expressed 'serious doubts about the ethical aspects' of the research and called for more studies on monkeys to prove that the procedure would be safe in humans. However, the fertility drugs the team had used successfully with their patients did not activate female primates very well and the few eggs, if any, they retrieved could not be fertilised in vitro. What they had hoped was possible in humans proved to be impossible in primates, yet they would receive no funding until they could demonstrate that IVF worked with monkeys. They were caught in a maddening catch-22 situation.

'I felt sick reading that letter,' wrote Edwards. 'This opposition was wounding. I read it again and felt angry.' He realised that they would have to fund the research themselves, somehow.

But they had more than just funding to worry about, finding themselves fiercely attacked on ethical, religious and political grounds too. At a conference of leading bioethical experts at the Kennedy Center in Washington DC, in a scheduled debate titled 'Fabricated Babies', Edwards defended IVF while Leon Kass, a biologist turned ethicist, and Paul Ramsey, the Princeton professor of religious studies, opposed it. Between them sat James Watson, the Nobel Prize-winning biologist. Having co-discovered the DNA double helix a decade earlier, he was a celebrity and someone with great influence over the public.

In the debate, Kass described IVF as 'a new holy war against human nature' that would lead to 'the divorce of the generation of new human life from human sexuality and ultimately from the confines of the human body'. He warned of ectogenesis – growing babies 'from sperm to term' in the laboratory – while Ramsey called IVF a 'disastrous further step toward the evil design of manufacturing our posterity'. The Princeton academic felt the technology to be such a danger to society that he said he hoped the first test-tube baby would be born so deformed and badly damaged that the entire enterprise would be brought to an immediate halt. Understandably, the audience were shocked at what they were hearing.

Another criticism held that IVF was neither a cure nor treatment for infertility. 'Without curing that condition, in vitro fertilisation concentrates on a product,' Ramsey said. 'It is therefore manufacture by biological technology, not medicine.' Instead of curing infertility, he argued, they were just giving an infertile woman a baby. But Edwards found the argument ridiculous.

'So much medical treatment is directed towards replacing a deficiency rather than producing a cure,' he said, using the examples of insulin for diabetes and spectacles for poor eyesight. Neither of those things *cured* the patient's condition, but they helped them live a better quality of life, and there was a role in medicine for that too, he argued.

'You can only go ahead with your work if you accept the necessity of infanticide,' Watson chimed in, addressing Edwards directly. 'There are going to be a lot of mistakes. What are we going to do with the mistakes?'

These words were powerful and petrifying to the public and scientists alike. No one knew what the first baby conceived in vitro would turn out like.

Three years later, at a congressional committee, Watson's scaremongering only got worse. 'All hell will break loose, politically and morally, all over the world,' he said. While some scientists worried it might be a slippery slope to genetically modified humans or babies grown entirely in labs, the press and public seemed more concerned at the prospect of human cloning. Terrible 'Brave New World visions' like these irritated Edwards. 'They are based on the pessimistic assumption that the worst will happen,' he wrote. 'The whole edifice of their argument is fragile – that nuclear physics led inevitably to the atom bomb, electricity to the electric chair, civil engineering to gas chambers. Surely acceptance of the beginning does not necessitate embracing undesirable ends?'

Edwards explained to the press over and over again that they just wanted to help people to have the families they wished for – families that they themselves had – children who were loved, adored, easily begotten. 'I was blessed,' he wrote. 'Patrick was blessed, some of our most stringent critics were fortunate to have children of their own. It was a priceless asset. It was a gift, the relationship of parent to a developing human being. And almost within our grasp was the possibility of passing on this gift to couples who had suffered years of childlessness and frustration.'

Edwards' empathy was clear. He was more than a physician trying to fix a clinical problem, he was a husband and father of five daughters; philosophically he understood what these families were missing out on. But more than that, he felt it was a human right. 'The Declaration of Human Rights made by the United Nations,' he wrote, 'included the right to establish a family.'

Before they married, John and Sandra had agreed they wanted children, just not yet. They decided to wait until they were thirty, after they'd seen the world and enjoyed life as a couple first. And that's what they did. For nearly three years they travelled around Australia, John finding work as a joiner and Sandra getting odd jobs in factories and for animal charities. They survived a cyclone that devastated Darwin on Christmas Eve, 1974. They adopted a stray cat, lost him in the storm, then found him again and brought him back to England. On their way home they visited Singapore, Hong Kong, Thailand, Burma, Nepal and Greece.

By the late 1970s, they were settled back in England and buying their first house. Sandra had been on the contraceptive pill for six years, but it was giving her head-splitting migraines. Although doctors had prescribed her the highest dose of painkillers available, it wasn't enough to ease the crunching headaches. She was left with an exasperating decision between head and womb, but she was only twenty-six and they weren't ready for a family yet. She picked up the phone and dialled the number of the family planning centre to order a different form of contraception that might alleviate her headaches.

John grabbed the phone out of her hand.

'Don't worry,' he said. 'Just come off it.'

'What?' Sandra said.

'Just come off the pill, we'll be all right.'

On 16 July 1978, the front cover of the *Daily News* read, 'Test-Tube Death Trial to Open', and the following morning Doris and John Del Zio arrived to find the small courtroom teeming with reporters. One of them, Tabitha Powledge, described the trial as being like a 'soap opera', whose characters all knew they were performing. She would recall 'flashes of genuine coldness and humor, compassion and cruelty' throughout, but for others, such as Marantz Henig, the trial ultimately came down to two important questions: 'Whether the stuff in Shettles's test tube was or was not a baby and whether it should or should not have been destroyed.'

One of the defence witnesses, Georgiana Jagiello, a professor of reproductive endocrinology, believed not only that no embryo would have resulted from the mixture that resembled 'chocolate milkshake' but that implanting it into Doris's uterus would have endangered her life, risking infection. Jagiello said that in her experience test tubes did not work as well for fertilisation as flat Petri dishes and the test-tube stopper Shettles had used was likely to have emitted fumes that killed the eggs. In order to keep the solution at the correct pH, the incubator would have required a mechanism that regulated the flow of carbon dioxide, which it did not. In other words, the 'baby' in the test tube was merely a mush of lifeless cells that never stood a chance. Then came the ethical considerations. No child had ever been conceived like this before, so there was no telling if test-tube babies were destined to be abnormal. No one knew if it was even possible to create life in this way.

When Doris Del Zio took the stand she broke down and wept. The jury saw the sad face of a thirty-four-year-old woman who simply wanted a baby and heard how her chance to do so, however tiny the odds, had been cruelly taken away from her without her consent. So who was to blame? 'If members of the jury ended up tossing a coin,' Powledge wrote, 'one could not exactly fault them.'

But on the seventh day of the trial, an extraordinary thing happened. News arrived at the courtroom that a baby had been born in Britain. Her name was Louise Brown and she had been conceived using in vitro fertilisation after ten years of trial and error by the British team: Steptoe, Edwards and Purdy. She was a happy, healthy and perfectly normal baby. The Del Zios and their legal team were delighted, while the defence were aghast. The judge quickly told the courtroom that the birth across the ocean was unrelated and instructed the jury in no uncertain terms to ignore it. But, Powledge wrote, 'it is hard to imagine that Louise Brown's birth mid-trial didn't strengthen the Del Zios' case.' It was a lightning bolt of serendipitous timing.

Three weeks later, the jury retired to consider their verdict. After a day of deliberation, they ruled in favour of the Del Zios, but the $1.5 million damages was deemed excessive. The jury awarded what it believed was more proportionate compensation: $50,000 to Doris and $3 to her husband John for the role he played.

The Del Zios may have won the case, but it didn't change the fact that they had not gone home with a baby. While it was a landmark trial and the first of its kind in the world, the ethics around the practising of IVF were still in contention. 'Did it make any new law, useful or not?' asked Powledge. 'Did it help us with the question of what to do about test tube babies? No and no.'

By the late 1970s many people were talking about test-tube babies around their dinner tables, but a trove of unanswered questions remained. When did an embryo become a baby? What rights did an embryo have? What should we do with excess embryos? Fifty years later, many Americans are still asking these same questions.

When Sandra and John read the news about 'Lovely Louise', they thought it was amazing but paid little attention. Louise's birth gave hope to thousands of couples who couldn't conceive naturally, but after less than a year of trying, John and Sandra did not yet realise that would include them.

In the years before they hailed Louise Brown as 'the Baby of the Century', the same newspapers had been filled with horror stories about assisted reproduction. Sandra's mother thought the technology was abhorrent and evil; she was staunchly against IVF and told them so. Sandra and John would never tell her that it was the same technology that brought her own grandchildren into the world.

Donor

Definition

1. A person who gives or donates
2. A person who gives part of their body to someone else

When the Medical Research Council refused funding for Edwards, Steptoe and Purdy to forge ahead with their IVF research, they did all they could to carry on, but times were bleak. They lost access to the hospital where they were working and had to settle somewhere much smaller that wasn't set up for their lab work.

'We needed more money to introduce sterile air, washable walls, clean surfaces, microscopes, balances, incubators, all the accoutrements needed for culturing embryos,' Edwards wrote. 'Patrick bought some of his equipment himself – operating tables and so on – but how we could have done with State funds!'

Then, one day, Edwards received a call from an American phone number. A woman in California had read about their work in a newspaper and wanted to help.

'Now here's the ironic thing,' he wrote. 'The publicity that had irritated us so much suddenly worked in our favour: it attracted private supporters to our cause, generous individuals, mostly American.'

The woman would give them the money under just one condition: she wanted to remain anonymous during her lifetime. When she died in 2014, at the age of ninety-three, her identity was finally revealed: her name was Lillian Lincoln Howell.

'This work would not have been possible without the generous benefaction of an American millionairess,' Edwards wrote, 'who herself suffered problems similar to those of the patients now being treated.' Between 1968 and 1978 she donated today's equivalent of around half a million pounds, providing a lifeline for the future of IVF. It may have been the British who gave birth to the first IVF baby, but we have the Americans to thank for funding it.

In early 2020, I was at work when I received a flurry of messages from my half-sisters, Libby and Lucy.

> It's happened! We found him!

OMG. Can you get a pic!?

> I'm emailing and asking yes.

> Will copy you in but not Bex as she needs to process!

Yes!!

Less than a year after I had discovered that I was donor-conceived, the sperm donor had signed up to the same DNA website and we were matched. I couldn't believe it.

Lucy messaged him and he replied straight away. She sent us a screenshot:

> Hi Lucy, from the results I have received today it appears that I am your biological father and also your twin sister Libby. I studied for my PhD at the University of Nottingham. Here is my email. I hope you have had an interesting life.

He had included his email address and signed off with his name. I panicked. He had the exact same name as my brother's friend's dad. Please don't let it be him, I whispered to myself. It would be so weird if my family knew him already. I quickly wrote a reply on the group chat.

Omg guys, I have just skimmed this. I'm at work.
Literally been following a police case for 16 hours straight and heading into a crime scene so can't deal with this right now but will chat later.

I was working on a television series about police detectives and we were in the middle of filming a big case that required all hands on deck. I had just pulled up to the house where the crime had taken place and was waiting for the scenes of crime officers to arrive. I set up the camera and tripod, ready to record, while frantically rereading Libby and Lucy's messages and googling the donor's name.

Two hours later, Lucy forwarded some photos the donor had sent of himself when he was younger. Phew. It wasn't the family friend. They had scraped a few more facts from his profile, including his birth year, revealing that he had been in his early twenties when he donated, and Lucy had also asked him some questions. He had a twenty-year-old daughter of his own, he said. His mother studied psychology, just like one of the twins in St Petersburg. Twins? Russia? Apparently we had international half-siblings too. It was a lot to take in.

Lucy asked him why he'd donated and whether he'd thought about it much in the years since.

'I am a chemist,' he replied, 'so to me the DNA that I provided is like some of the software programming, while the rest of the software and hardware (the egg) is provided by the mother. If a couple are willing to go through IVF then that would surely mean a loving home and a good nurturing environment for a child to grow up in.'

I felt comforted by this. He knew my parents would be good parents. He knew that what he provided was a gift.

Libby sent a picture of the profile photo attached to his email address. He looked a bit like my dad when he was younger. Libby and Lucy said he didn't look anything like their dad.

Aside from four hours of sleep, I had been working for forty-eight hours in a row, having to wash my underwear in a hotel sink with hand soap at 2 a.m. because there was no time to get back home to change. The next evening I was finally on the train back to London.

> I haven't processed any of this as I've not had time. Just had a beer on the train and it's finally kicking in. How crazy that this has all happened?!?!!! I honestly did not believe we would ever know who he was.

Libby and Lucy now had an email chain with him and were asking lots of questions. Everything from 'What's your favourite cocktail?' to 'Is your second toe longer than your big toe?' I was still in shock. It felt like a step too far to contact him myself and I'm not sure there was anything else I needed to know since they were already giving him the full Spanish inquisition. Luckily, he didn't seem to mind.

Labour

Definition

1. Physical work
2. The last stage of pregnancy in which a baby is born
3. A political party in the UK

I was watching a woman give birth on all fours in her living room. The curtains were closed and two midwives in purple uniforms lingered nearby. It was 2021 and I was filming for a BBC documentary series about home birth, and the 5 a.m. call from the midwife had me clambering out of bed and into the car with my camera kit.

It wasn't ideal that this was my first time meeting Katherine, in actual labour, but the on-call filming rota had its inevitable faults. After the pandemic lockdowns had ended, I left London and relocated to Yorkshire to work on the series. That morning I drove the forty minutes from Leeds to Katherine's home near Bradford, hoping she wouldn't mind a stranger being the one to film her birth. Fortunately, when I arrived, Katherine and her mum Sue greeted me like an old friend.

'Come on in!' Sue chimed as I stepped inside the warm house. 'They said it might snow again,' she smiled, with the aspiration that her second grandchild might be born in a flurry of snowfall.

It was early December and the morning air was frosted with a sort of tenderness, that joyful anticipation that illuminates the atmosphere in the weeks before Christmas. I greeted the midwives, who I knew well by then, as they took Katherine's measurements, gently lifting her lace-frilled nightgown to one side. Then, a contraction. In the girdle of an earthy groan, Katherine paused, lifted her head and politely requested a glass of water. Labour was equal parts primal and delicate, I thought. I asked Katherine if she was happy for me to start filming and she said yes.

It might not have been the best idea to work on a series about babies when I was feeling broody, and had been for years, but I'd hoped that seeing birth up close might put me off, or at least stall the engine, while I waited for my partner to catch up with my longing to hold a baby of our own. In reality, working on the series did the opposite; I craved the experience of pregnancy more than ever. Birth was real-life magic, one person becoming two. It was the most dignified thing I had ever seen. And, I learned, it could also be pretty funny. As her contractions raged on, Katherine cursed all men for ever daring to complain about being 'kicked in the knackers'.

'How dare they?' she fumed. 'They have it so bloody easy!'

We all nodded in agreement.

The television was on in the background and, in an attempt to keep things calm and festive, one of the midwives discreetly changed the channel to a snowy merry-go-round scene with plinky Christmas music. The room felt more tranquil at once, like we were inside a snow globe that had been shaken and was now settling down. A few minutes into this peaceful meditation, Katherine shouted:

'Turn off that shit!'

I tried to keep the camera still as I vibrated with laughter.

Throughout my six months of filming inside people's basements, birth pools and bathrooms, the mothers and midwives had shown me what a privilege it is to grow a human inside you. Turning parents' lives upside down and forcing them to reassemble it Lego brick by Lego brick. And yet, growing up I had never pushed around dolls or had any affinity for babies. I found them unpredictable, smelly and certainly not cute. Drooling, bald, poo machines. I didn't understand why people raved about having them so much.

I started taking the pill when I was fifteen and like most young women who came of age during the British government's anti-teenage pregnancy movement in the 2000s, I was terrified of accidentally getting pregnant. The Labour campaign, launched in 1999, aimed to halve under eighteens' conception rate within a decade – at 4.6 per cent it was one of the highest in Europe. The government strategy included improving sexual education in schools and accessibility to contraceptives, and providing more support for young parents to prevent further pregnancies. The national publicity campaign informed teenagers 'how hard it is to be a parent and how easy it is to get pregnant'. Within fifteen years, the teenage pregnancy rate had 'dropped like a stone' to 2.3 per cent and was being described as 'the success story of our time'.

In my school year of over a hundred girls, I don't think a single one gave birth before the age of twenty-six. Five years later, I'd estimate still only a third have. It's taken me decades to shake off the intrinsic fear associated with the word 'pregnant' and the notion that missing a pill might ruin my career prospects forever.

My parents did not want us to have children before we were ready, but they also knew how precarious procreation could be. My dad once told my sister and me that if we were to fall pregnant by accident, he didn't want us to get an abortion.

Today the teenage pregnancy rate in Britain is the lowest on record and 72 per cent lower than in the 1990s. But it isn't just the rate of teenage pregnancies that has gone down: all pregnancy rates have. These days, new mothers are skewing older and having fewer children. The average age of a first-time mother is now thirty-two, the oldest since records began and more than ten years older than my parents' generation. For the first time ever, more people are turning thirty without children than with, and the average number of children per family has fallen below two. Is it a coincidence or did the government campaign a generation ago somewhat backfire? Ironically, various groups are now campaigning for a more balanced approach to sex education in schools, including giving information about the best time to conceive, how lifestyle factors affect fertility, and the limits of IVF and egg freezing.

There are other reasons, of course, why my generation is not popping out babies like we used to. An emphasis on careers (too often incompatible with childcare), endless financial crashes and cost-of-living crises, unaffordable housing, app-swiping singledom and concerns about climate change have shaped a generation of men and women who do not feel ready for the responsibility of another human, or have decided to forgo parenthood altogether.

Like many people, I naively assumed that in my mid-to-late twenties I would buy a house, get married and then children would come along in due course. While some friends and family have done just that, for me, now thirty-three and in my fourth long-term relationship, I find myself unmarried, childless and renting despite having a good career, earning a good wage and having been in good relationships with good men. So far, so good, yet I find myself adrift of the formal adult commitments we were told were waiting for us, and it seems I'm not the only one. Such markers of 'success' are slowly coming undone as property ownership, marriage and birth rates are all at a record low. Many of us are re-evaluating our relationship with them, through choice or otherwise. For some these traditional markers of 'achievement' are out of reach for financial reasons, but I sense there is an emotional gap too.

Having children is the only one of these milestones that is truly time-sensitive, but not one of the men I've been in long-term, committed relationships with in my twenties or thirties has been 'ready' for children. They assured me that they wanted to be with me and that they definitely wanted children, just 'not yet'. Okay, I said, stayed on the pill and waited. That was all fine, except for one thing that kept nagging at me. Something I couldn't ignore any more. Stabbing pains on the toilet and during sex, brain fog, fatigue, bloating. I genuinely thought these things happened to every woman, we just didn't talk about it. And then there were the 'waterfalls'; dramatic stories of my torrential bleeding had entertained my friends for years. As a teenager I had soaked entire pairs of trousers, ruined bedsheets and stained car seats through three layers of clothing. Occasionally I bled through tampons, sanitary pads and underwear all at the same time. I didn't understand how I could lose so much blood and still be standing. My monthly cycle required military-level preparation and planning, and yet my bleeding was irregular so I never knew when it would happen. Throughout school, university and my early working life I never left the house without supplies in my bag and would feel anxious if I didn't know where the nearest toilet was. But they were just 'heavy periods', no one ever mentioned anything else. When a friend told me she only bled a teaspoon every month, I started to wonder, why was I bleeding buckets?

One day I'd had enough. I'd been bleeding for a few days already so before work I put a tampon in. It was 2018 and I was filming an interview with two men – an actor and a rugby player – and a male camera assistant, when I felt the sudden, familiar flood. I panicked but couldn't let it show on my face. We had just started recording; I felt paralysed. I was the director and main camera operator – I couldn't just leave while the two men were in the flow of conversation. I dared not look down in case my jeans had turned from blue to red, like a boiled lobster. It was that hot pulse of humiliation again. I stood there for another thirty minutes, waiting for an appropriate break, then darted to the toilet. Thankfully the damage was mostly contained; my pale blue jeans were thick enough to keep the stains to the inside. I stuffed a clump of toilet paper into my underwear and walked back out, ready for the next take.

But inside I was furious. This unpredictable nonsense was seeping into my professional life too. I was angry that archaic societal taboos had made me feel unable to speak up with the men in the room. Men who didn't have to put up with sporadic uncontrollable gushing from their genitals during work hours. But deep down I knew that women shouldn't have to put up with it either.

On the train back from the shoot I texted my mum, who was sympathetic and suggested that, like her, I might have something called endometriosis.

> I've been randomly bleeding very heavily for no reason including in the middle of filming just now
>
> Don't ignore the bleeding !!
>
> And the worst thing is that I was already wearing a super tampon!!
>
> You need a trip to the doctor.
>
> Wear a skirt/dress and an old fashioned sanitary towel as well as your tampon
>
> Did you have heavy periods when you were younger? Was it a symptom of your endometriosis?
>
> Yes I did but only when my monthly's were due and I had really bad pain (didn't know it was worse than other girls until I was diagnosed)
>
> Yeah that's the thing, you don't know any different

> But apparently being on the pill helped me without realising.
>
> Make a GP appointment
>
> People don't understand how traumatising it can be. I would be nearing panic attacks if I didn't know where the nearest toilet was at uni and have carried sanitary products in my bag pretty much everyday for the past 10 years
>
> No wonder you're tired constantly.
>
> You're wanting a family in the future so it's really important.
>
> I had surgery to remove it but it was too late as my fallopian tubes were blocked and stuck. Don't ignore it until you want to start a family like I did. You are older now than when I started investigations.

I googled endometriosis.
Endometriosis is an inflammatory condition where tissue, similar to the lining of the womb, grows outside it in other parts of the body.
Mum had been diagnosed with stage four endometriosis, the most severe stage, at the age of twenty-eight. I was already twenty-seven by then and had been ignoring the symptoms for years. For Sandra, the endometrial tissue had blocked her fallopian tubes, making it impossible for egg and sperm to meet. The first symptom she became aware of was not being able to get pregnant. The other symptoms she had thought were just a normal part of being a woman. It's amazing what we put up with in ignorance.

The next day I called my GP with a list of symptoms. Perhaps because I'm an articulate white woman, I was lucky to be taken seriously straight away and referred to a specialist, but I know this is not always the case and many women are ignored, gaslit or misdiagnosed. Long waiting lists don't make the process any easier. Globally, the average wait time for an endometriosis diagnosis is seven years; in the UK it's nearly nine years.

A few months later, I was given a date for a laparoscopy: abdominal keyhole surgery. My consultant told me that endometriosis is found in only 50 per cent of such surgeries. I suddenly worried that I'd caused all this fuss for nothing and imagined how embarrassed I'd feel if they didn't find anything.

On the day of the operation, Sam was slumped beside me. We had hosted a drag-themed Halloween party the evening before and he was feeling its after-effects. 'HallowQueen' had been in the calendar before my surgery date and I refused to let anything interrupt my social plans. I loved how Sam encouraged my crazy ideas (often involving fancy dress), enjoyed hosting at our flat and always made sure everyone had a drink. As something of a musical genius, he often entertained our friends with his keyboard or guitar, taking requests and playing any song by ear, beautifully. But being the life and soul of the party also has its downsides.

I didn't drink any alcohol but everyone else did, including Sam. As I lay in the hospital bed at 8 a.m. nervously waiting to be wheeled in, he was curled up in the foetal position on the chair next to me. We'd been in a relationship for two and a half years by then. He was thirty – three years older than me – but adamant he didn't want children any time soon. Maybe in ten years, he said, though I never knew if he was being serious or not. *Starting a family at the age of forty, surely not?*

When I returned from the operating table, the consultant explained that he'd found endometriosis lesions all over my bladder, bowels and womb. Finally a reason for everything. I was relieved to know that I hadn't been making it all up. He said there was no sign of endometriosis on my ovaries and fallopian tubes, for now – which was good news for my fertility – and he had cauterised as much as he could so it should hopefully relieve my symptoms.

I video-called my parents to let them know, but I could barely speak. The breathing tubes inserted during the surgery had left my throat so dry the words seemed to disappear as I was saying them. I was trying to be strong and let Mum and Dad know I was fine but was literally choking on every other word. I sounded like I was about to burst into tears. I kept trying, but it got worse. Eventually the frustration of not being able to express myself and the weight of saying the diagnosis out loud for the first time did make me cry. A raspy sob that hurt my windpipe. My parents stared back at the screen in silence. They've never been good with emotions and clearly didn't know what to say. It must have reminded them of their own journey; of surgery and sedation, new medical terms and unanswerable questions. Treatments without cures. I was reliving some of their pain, and there was nothing they could do about it.

A little while later the surgeon came back into the room. 'Do you want children?' he asked us.

'Yes, one day,' I replied.

'Okay, well you should do it sooner rather than later. Ideally in the next couple of years.'

Panic latched on to Sam's face. This was not part of his plan. But I was pleased. It meant there was more than just me encouraging the idea – a doctor was suggesting it too, and a man, no less. Maybe he would listen to him.

The consultant left the room and I turned towards Sam.

'Okay fine, let's say five years rather than ten,' he said.

I nodded, but I was forlorn. The doctor said sooner. My body might not wait five years. Then Sam made a joke about starting right there and then, in the hospital bed. His sister and brother-in-law were trying for their second child and he joked that we could try and beat them to it. But obviously that's all it was, a joke.

Over the next couple of years, I thought about our timeline for having children a lot, but every time I wanted to bring it up with Sam I stopped myself, not wanting to scare him off or make him feel pressured. I was still in my twenties after all, plenty of time, but I couldn't stop replaying a conversation we'd had early on in our relationship, one that was stamped into my memory.

We'd been dating for almost a year and things were good. It was a hot day in June and we were strolling around the canal paths in Little Venice, near to where I lived with three friends: Emma, Annabeth and Joyce. The four of us shared the ground-floor apartment of a red-brick terraced mansion in Maida Vale. To make the rent cheaper we had turned the living room into a bedroom, making do with a sofa in the kitchen as a small communal space. We were such good friends anyway that we spent time in each other's bedrooms, catching up, laughing, strewn across our beds like sisters.

Emma and Annabeth were friends from university and Joyce was a school friend of Annabeth's. We were in our early to mid-twenties, enjoying all that our fledgling careers in London had to offer. We all worked in Soho: Emma and I in TV production, Annabeth as a model and Joyce in an upmarket café, bringing home leftovers of pesto chicken breast and cherry-chocolate brownies. We sometimes brought home Tinder dates too, as always at least one of us was single and dating. It was our *Friends* or *Girls* era. We watched the Spice Girls movie, made pancakes in our pyjamas and one year got so excited about Christmas we decorated the tree in mid-November. The four of us lived there for three years and I loved it. Sometimes we imagined our futures, speculating about who would get married and have children first.

As Sam and I wandered along the canal path, life felt good and the future promising. I was excelling at my career in TV, getting to travel around the world, and I felt happy with how our relationship was going. Everything seemed to be falling into place. Sam had the option to return to Toronto after twelve months of working in his firm's London office, but because things were going so well he decided to apply for an extension to his work visa. We had even discussed getting a marriage visa instead.

'I need to call my mom and let her know that I'm staying in the UK for another year,' Sam said. 'I might call her now.'

'She'll probably think I'm pregnant and you're staying forever,' I laughed.

'Don't joke about that,' he said, his voice changing. 'It's not funny to joke about getting someone pregnant.'

I was taken aback. 'Oh. Okay. I'm definitely not pregnant by the way, I was just joking.'

'I can't think of anything worse that could happen right now,' he said.

'Wait, what?' I said, then paused. 'You can't imagine *anything* worse than me getting pregnant?'

'Pretty much.'

I stopped walking. I realised he was deadly serious.

'But why?' I asked, confused. 'You're twenty-eight and I'm twenty-five, it's not like we're teenagers.'

'It would be terrible timing, I don't even live here permanently.'

'I know, but we would figure it out. We're in a stable relationship, we both have good jobs. We'd be fine,' I said. 'Obviously it wouldn't be ideal, but surely it's not the absolute worst thing you can imagine?'

'It's pretty high up there,' he said.

I was stunned, a couple of notches from heartbroken. He seemed genuinely devastated at the concept of having a child with me, his long-term girlfriend.

But I knew timings were important to him. Working in his

world required rigid planning, watertight schedules, perfect execution and an agreed exchanging of contracts. Certainly no mistakes, that was crucial. This was the language he spoke. Or perhaps it was the language all men spoke, I wasn't sure. Either way, it was at this relatively early stage of our relationship that I realised we were on different pages. I didn't want children immediately, maybe in the next few years, but the idea of nudging someone from 'worst-imaginable-scenario' to 'over-the-moon-with-joy' at your pregnancy seemed unlikely in that timeframe. A seed of sadness took root in my belly.

I was on the pill and so an 'accident' was incredibly unlikely, but I wondered, did I even want children with someone who felt this way about an unplanned pregnancy? The way he spoke felt like a verbal warning. Whatever you do, don't get pregnant. Don't forget your pill. Don't ruin my life. The responsibility of being female felt heavier. The possibility of motherhood shifted further away.

When I recounted this story to a friend recently, she said that an old boyfriend once told her that if she got pregnant he would push her down the stairs. It was a joke, apparently. Perhaps these kinds of jokes would be more funny if violence against women and girls was less prevalent in our society; if it wasn't now considered a 'national emergency' in the UK. But the reality is that women are often threatened or punished by the men who could (or do) get them pregnant. Blamed for their biology, punished for growing a seed planted by someone else. Such hostile attitudes – in place of taking responsibility for the potential consequences of their actions – make procreation (and sex at all) an even more delicate subject for women to navigate, and one that might compromise their safety. What strikes me the most is that these were responses from men in long-term, loving relationships. Not one-night stands or casual hook-ups or rape. These were men who were supposed to be our teammates and allies in the world. Yet their words – laced with belligerence and lacking in support for their partner and any potential child – felt not just like red flags for our romantic futures but like a deep betrayal of friendship.

I was shocked at what my friend told me. I felt sad for her younger self who had to question the validity of a physical threat disguised as a joke by a partner who apparently loved her. How many young women, I wonder, are told in no uncertain terms that pregnancy is a *terrible* thing and if it happens they are the ones at fault. Contraception is a physical, emotional and often invisible labour handed to women from a young age. We are expected to endure the hormonal side effects of the contraceptive pill, implant, patch, IUD or injection, or to seek out and ingest the morning after pill within hours of sex if barrier forms of contraception fail. Since no form of contraception is perfect, sexual intercourse always carries a risk, however small, of pregnancy. The responsibility is always carried by women, despite 100 per cent of unwanted pregnancies being caused by men. As author Gabrielle Blair put it so deftly: ovulation is involuntary, ejaculation is not.

A couple of years after the don't-get-pregnant conversation with Sam, we had moved in together and were enjoying the inner-city lifestyle that London had to offer. Sam had insisted we live in central London and I agreed, on the condition that we moved further out in a couple of years. He loved drinking Old Fashioneds and staying out until the early hours with work colleagues or taking friends to his favourite 'dive bar', rammed with sweaty bodies every Saturday night. These things were freedom to him, and for over ten years I liked that kind of carefree lifestyle too. But by my late twenties I was getting bored. I felt like our weekends lacked meaning; they were just a drinking-hangover cycle on repeat. We lived a stone's throw from Liverpool Street, the busiest railway station in Britain, so we were well located for everything London had to offer, but I also felt suffocated by tourists, litter and pollution. After two years in our flat, I desperately wanted to move out of London, or at least to the suburbs where we could afford a garden and an extra bedroom for a child. Sam agreed to look at houses elsewhere, but I knew he wanted our lives to stay the same for a few more years. The same years that doctors told me I didn't have.

Occasionally I asked Sam what he wanted his future to look like, hoping it would involve some mention of children among career ambitions and travelling the world. He said he saw himself as an old man at a table full of children and grandchildren and I was relieved.

'I want to be the head of the family,' he said. 'Sat at the end of the table, like my grandad was.'

I was glad to hear this, but over time I realised he seemed more interested in the notion of having *had* a family than the reality of actually raising one. Sam loved his niece and nephews but repeatedly complained about a specific time he'd witnessed his sister changing a foul-smelling nappy in the middle of a street on a hot day. He seemed physically repulsed by some of the more undesirable but necessary stages of parenting, and it concerned me.

In the end it didn't matter. Two years later we broke up, no closer to having children and never having really discussed it again properly.

Back in Bradford, after three hours and several cups of tea, the midwives let me know that the birth was imminent. Katherine had been manoeuvring her body into different positions around the room, trying to get comfortable. Eventually she positioned herself in front of the Christmas tree, a gaudy circus of plastic, adorned in eighties tinsel. The Nativity scene was set. She was Mary and the midwives were the wise women, bringing gifts of pain relief, moral support and goodwill. Perhaps I was the donkey, observing: bemused, humbled.

As I filmed Katherine giving birth in her living room, the surgeon's words echoed in my mind. I was thirty years old and it had been three years since my diagnosis. Katherine had also turned thirty recently and was lamenting not being able to drink on a big birthday again, since she'd also been pregnant with her first child on her twenty-first birthday. Two kids before thirty was totally normal, I reasoned, so why did it feel like I was crazy for wanting my first child now? Most of the women I filmed on the series were younger than me, some by more than a decade, others by just a few years but on their second or third child. Even one of my filming colleagues was heavily pregnant. Babies were no longer in my peripheral vision but blinding and unbearable at times. Every pregnancy announcement, baby shower or toddler milestone felt bittersweet. Good for them. How lucky they were to have found someone ready to be a parent at the same time. Why did talking about children with my partner feel like stepping on eggshells? Were all men so hesitant or was I just unlucky? Maybe the problem was me.

In Katherine's living room, a kind of radiance surrounded us; perhaps it was maternal love. Despite us taking over his home, Katherine's husband had stayed largely out of the way – he was supportive of the filming but not keen on the cameras himself. This moment, therefore, was a time for documenting the strength of women: Katherine, and the astonishing power of her body, and the midwives and their remarkable intuition honed by expertise and experience. All captured by myself and another female colleague who joined us as the birth began. A team of fiercely patient women, ready to welcome another into the world.

Kneeling over the sofa, Katherine gave one last push. But when the baby girl arrived, she was silent. One of the midwives rubbed her little back and spoke to her with such gentle reassurance that my eyes welled up.

'You're a bit surprised, aren't you?'

Nothing. Time suspended. I panicked, camera still rolling.

'Are you gonna give us a big shout?' the midwife continued, calmly.

The room was still. Please be okay, we uttered, a chorus of silent prayer. *Please be okay.*

Birth must be a shock, leaving a warm cosy haven for an exposing world of senses and utter sovereignty. I felt for this tiny, precious baby. It was all too much.

Still nothing, just torrential silence.

Then the little girl let out an enormous scream. Finally she was ready to speak.

Wanted

Definition

1. Wished for
2. Searched for by the police because of a crime

By 1983, John and Sandra had been trying to conceive for six years with no luck. In the meantime they were rearing puppies. Sandra had trained as a dog groomer and John had built the kennels for her to run her business from, while he worked as a self-employed joiner. Their Old English sheepdog, Candy, had recently given birth to ten puppies. One was stillborn and they kept one, so there were eight puppies left to sell. When the puppies were a few weeks old, a woman and her teenage son came to choose one. The following week, Sandra called the family to give them an update about the collection date. A teenage girl answered the phone.

'Hello. Is your mum or brother there?' Sandra asked. 'Could I speak to one of them?'

A few hours later, the girl walked to her boyfriend's house just over a mile away, but she never arrived. The police were called and family and friends began searching for her. The next morning, her brother found her naked body dumped in a nearby field.

Eight months later, the murder of sixteen-year-old Colette Aram became the first case ever to be shown on the BBC series *Crimewatch*. Despite hundreds of tip-offs after the television appeal, detectives still had no suspect. It would become one of the largest and longest manhunts in police history.

And yet there was plenty of evidence. There were eyewitnesses: the killer had approached two other girls before abducting Aram at knife-point and dragging her into the back of a stolen car. After murdering Colette, the man walked into a pub nearby and ordered a drink and sandwich. The barmaid noticed he had blood on his hands before he went to the toilet and wiped them clean. When she saw Aram's murder on the news the next day, she collected a paper towel from the toilet bin and notified the police who identified blood and semen on it. But that was as far as forensic testing went at the time. They had the murderer's DNA, but no way to track him down.

In 2004, *Crimewatch* ran the story again for its twentieth anniversary show. By then the police had managed to build a DNA profile of the killer using modern cutting-edge forensic technology, but they found no match on the national database. Four years later, a man was arrested on a motoring offence and his DNA swab provided a close match to the blood on the paper towel. There was just one problem: he hadn't been born at the time of Colette Aram's death, so detectives arrested his father, fifty-year-old Paul Hutchinson, instead, and charged him with murder. He was sentenced to life with a minimum of twenty-five years. Eighteen months later, he killed himself in prison.

When Colette's brother came to collect the puppy, Sandra and John didn't know what to say. Like everyone else, they had been following the murder investigation on the news, horrified that something like this could happen in their local area.

When my parents told me the story, aside from feeling the heartache of a young woman's life senselessly extinguished too soon, I was fascinated by the concept that future technology – incomprehensible in the present – could be capable of solving murders from the past. It's like a form of time travel and I find the idea comforting: that the truth is inescapable and that justice will, eventually, prevail.

When we were eleven years old, Mum and Dad sat us all down for a 'talk'. It was the don't-take-candy-from-strangers talk.

'Don't get into a car with anyone you don't know,' they said. 'Even if they tell you they're friends with your parents and were sent to come and get you. Even if they say your mum is in hospital. Even if it's a woman who seems nice. Whatever they say, don't trust them.'

But it's hard to know who to trust sometimes. The 'talk' was fuelled by a story that was dominating the news at the time. Two girls, the same age as us, called Holly and Jessica, had been murdered by their school caretaker. His girlfriend, the girls' teaching assistant, had helped cover his tracks and provided an alibi. I understood 'stranger danger', but what about caretakers or teaching assistants or teachers? What about police officers or doctors or swim coaches? As a child, the rules weren't very clear. As an adult, they still aren't. A few years ago, while I was making a BBC documentary with the police about historically low rape convictions, a woman called Sarah Everard was raped and murdered by a police officer.

From a young age I've felt a pull towards the psychologically darker sides of life. At school, while the other twelve-year-old children were writing stories about aliens and magic, I wrote one about a child in a coma, lying in a hospital bed flanked by her parents who were in the throes of a divorce. My teacher read it aloud to the class and my parents still have a copy of it. I'm not sure if they were proud or concerned. Looking back, I wonder if the news stories that punctuated my childhood had anything to do with why I became a documentary filmmaker. Looking into the eyes of murderers, consoling the families of victims, interrogating the justice system.

A few months ago, I asked my mum if they were offered counselling during the sperm donation process. Yes, she said, they had one counselling session.

'Can you tell me about it?'

'I remember the counsellor looked at John and said: "How are you going to feel knowing that your wife has another man's sperm inside of her?"'

I gasped in disbelief.

'That got his back up straight away,' Mum said.

'Bloody hell. They didn't need to phrase it like that.'

'I know. I guess they wanted to check that he really was okay with it and wouldn't back out later on.'

My aunt – and godmother – once told my parents that she thought using a sperm donor was like committing adultery. My dad has never forgotten it. No doubt there are still many people around the world who feel this way.

Thou shalt not commit adultery is number seven of the Ten Commandments in the Bible. We still say 'commit' because until 1857 it was considered a crime in the UK, punishable by whipping, branding or prison. Surprisingly, adultery is still technically illegal in more than a dozen US states.

My parents wanted children and that is not a crime.

Six weeks after the initial conversation with my parents about being donor-conceived, I was back home, sitting in the living room with Dad. He was in his armchair, like usual, watching the news on TV, when a strapline appeared onscreen: DOCTOR PATERNITY SCANDAL. A Dutch fertility doctor had used his own sperm to impregnate hundreds of patients without their consent. I froze. Dad and I sat there in silence. We hadn't talked about the family secret since the day it came to light and it felt so awkward to be confronted with not just sperm donation but an illicit, darker side of it. The news segment seemed to go on forever and I willed it to end. When it finally did, neither of us said anything. The odds were that I wasn't conceived by a dodgy doctor, though I couldn't be sure.

In the last decade there has been such a swell of documentaries about sperm donation 'gone wrong' that it has practically formed its own true crime genre. From serial sperm donors who have hundreds of children to doctors who secretly use their own sperm, the stories are chilling and consistently rank in streaming platforms' most popular shows. In the same way that modern technology has opened the door to con artists exploiting dating apps, the phenomenon of 'fertility fraud' is growing. It's not hard to understand why the fertility industry is susceptible to corruption and crime. Faced with a relatively new technology, lawmakers have been slow to keep up and many countries still have no laws or official regulations when it comes to fertility treatment. The clientele tend to be single women and couples who might be considered vulnerable. Often they have been trying to conceive for years, their options have narrowed and the biological clock is ticking. Similar to many new industries that once started from an act of altruism, capitalism has dug its claws in. Sperm and egg donation have become multi-million-dollar businesses; fertile ground for profit and ripe for exploitation.

I was reluctant to watch any of these documentaries; they felt both too distinct from my own story and too close to home. From a filmmaker's perspective, I also worried that the stories would be sensationalised and the children at their heart would be forgotten or further stigmatised. But I knew I should force myself to sit down and watch. If I was going to write about sperm donation I needed to face the subject head on and acknowledge the wider public context. I had to accept that many people's awareness of sperm donation these days arises through scandals like these.

In the case of the fertility doctors, some of the women in the documentaries had been sexually assaulted or raped in their doctor's office, but most were secretly inseminated without their consent. Often their partners had provided sperm samples and had assumed these were used, while others had been matched up with specific sperm donors and been told there would not be more than a handful of half-siblings for their child. When these children later signed up to DNA websites as adults, it came as a surprise to many to find they had dozens or even hundreds of half-siblings. And yet there were no laws that made it a crime. Legally, it was unprecedented territory. One of the adult children wondered how it was that she lived in a world where she could be charged for spitting in someone's face but the doctor – who masturbated then inseminated her mother with his own sperm without her consent – faced no charges at all.

At first each of the doctors denied any involvement, seemingly hoping it would all just blow over. Perhaps they had not appreciated that sperm become babies and babies become adults, with their own minds and consciences. It only took one strong-minded individual to start asking questions, recruit a mega-team of half-siblings and blow the whole house down.

Like me, many of the children had found out about the circumstances of their conception by innocently signing up to a DNA website. A birthday present or a Christmas gift that swiftly turned into an unexpected nightmare. Once you've unwrapped a hand grenade in your family's living room, you can't go back, you have to deal with the devastation.

So far, forty-five cases of fertility doctors inseminating their patients have been uncovered around the world, resulting in hundreds of children. For the children who do discover the truth – many will be unaware, having not signed up to a DNA website – there are support groups available, with various online communities for 'donor deceived' and 'doctor conceived' people springing up over the last ten years.

'I just felt bad for my mother. Here she was, you know, a young woman, she just wanted to have a family like anyone else,' says one of the doctor-conceived children. I have a great deal of sympathy for the families who find themselves in this cycle of torment. Is there any bigger breach of trust? Any worse misuse of authority? A form of abuse more enduring than one that lives on through the faces of your children and grandchildren?

The power dynamics involved in these cases are deeply troubling. We are supposed to trust doctors; they see us at our most vulnerable and undignified, so to have been not only abused by them but also the physical incubator of their own secret sick spawning game is an unimaginably complex scenario in which to find yourself. One woman discovered that she had been conceived this way after watching a TV show in which a handful of her half-siblings, who looked like her, were trying to take the doctor to court. To add insult to injury, the doctor was also her own OB-GYN doctor. He had examined her most intimate areas, fully aware that he was her biological father. It was a final twist of the knife.

My journey with deceit has been far less disturbing than for these families, but I believe that if there is any comfort to be had, it's in the knowledge that we were all deeply wanted. Indeed, the parents in the films are quick to affirm that their children are loved. The dynamics of their conception were regrettable but their children were not. As one mother put it: 'You can't be angry when you have what you always dreamed of.'

But many of them are angry. Some of the doctor-conceived adults have taken their biological fathers to court in an attempt to make them face justice for violating their mothers, all while knowing that they would not be here otherwise.

Some of the doctor-conceived children have inherited health conditions, noting that the doctors wouldn't have passed their own donor-screening programmes. All ninety-four of one American doctor's biological children have autoimmune conditions. One of them has Sjögren's syndrome, which means she can't produce saliva or tears. 'So you won't ever see me cry,' she says, movingly, in the courtroom. 'My tears have literally been taken away from me.'

If I've learned anything from making true crime documentaries, it's that as a society we are desperate to look into an 'evil' person's eyes and understand *why*. What made them do it? Was it their childhood? Could they be my neighbour, friend, husband? What kind of man would want to procreate with scores of different women? A narcissist? A megalomaniac? A misogynist? I have seen in my work that very few perpetrators of sexual abuse are remorseful; virtually none show any empathy towards their victims, and some even believe that what they did was good. The same seems to be true for fertility fraud. The doctors tended to actively avoid answering why, they simply sat back and quietly admired the army they had created.

With regards to the so-called 'super donors' – the men who decide to voluntarily donate on a mass scale – I was baffled watching them try to explain their motives. These men had often signed up to multiple sperm banks and unregulated websites at a time, ignoring any paperwork requiring them to declare if they were donating elsewhere and lying to recipients about the number of families they had previously donated to. As a result, some of them have offspring numbering in the seven or eight hundreds.

Louis, who used a pseudonym, tells us that he was abandoned by his father growing up. So far, so Freudian. But his motivation for donating, he says, was his own funeral.

'There's only one moment when it becomes clear how important you were to people. That is when your funeral is held,' he tells us. 'How many people will attend? The idea was, I would die sooner or later and who would say kind words at my funeral? Who would remember me? It became something of an obsession: I had to have offspring to arrange my funeral.'

To increase the odds of at least a few children tracking him down and attending his funeral, Louis donated sperm three times a week for seventeen years, resulting in approximately two hundred children. He admits it was a crazy idea, but it worked. He has formed a father-like relationship with a couple of the donor children and no doubt they will be there to wave off his coffin when the time comes. Others are not so forgiving. 'I felt like an overbred laboratory rat,' said one of his other biological children.

Louis also tells the filmmakers that he is probably autistic.

'I've always had trouble interacting with people,' he says. 'I don't enter into relationships, I don't have friends, or my friendships never lasted long. I did try to find a girlfriend by way of personal ads, but that didn't work. Then in the early 1980s, I read in a magazine about artificial insemination: "sperm bank short of donors". I thought, this is what I will do. This might be a way for me to get relatives after all.'

For Louis, being a donor was a way to live a 'normal' life that wasn't otherwise available to him. Having a wife and kids seemed out of reach, so he bypassed the usual social constructs and went straight to procreation. His honesty is refreshing, but the whole scenario is deeply unsettling.

'The cosmos gave me the chance to arrange this,' he says. 'I think our biggest fear in life is not to die but to be forgotten.'

One problem with having this many offspring is the risk of half-siblings inadvertently forming relationships. One of the children of the Dutch doctor matched with a woman on Tinder who he said looked 'just like one of his sisters'. He turned out to be right. It is the reason why many countries have a family limit per donor rule. In Spain it is capped at six families, Norway eight, Britain ten, Sweden twelve, Germany fifteen and the Netherlands twenty-five. In the United States there are guidelines but currently no legal limits on how many families can be created from each sperm donor. There is also no global or European database to check if donors are donating elsewhere. Apparently breeding cattle is more strictly regulated. For those men who decided to make donating their full-time job and committed themselves to tricking the system, the results were stupefying. The Netflix documentary *The Man with 1000 Kids* speaks for itself. Not only is the risk of consanguinity and accidental incest much higher for these children and their children, but it appears to be a 'biodiversity hazard' for the human species. A man with 500 children will have a staggering 15,000 descendants within 100 years.

Yet this isn't an entirely new phenomenon. While the most children a woman has ever given birth to is sixty-nine, for men the numbers are exponentially bigger. Genghis Khan springs to mind, but over the centuries more than thirty men are known to have had over one hundred children each, some of them many hundreds. Yet for most of human history, the number of mothers has always outnumbered fathers. While there is, of course, always one male and one female parent when a child is conceived, the number of women and men who have passed on their DNA throughout time has not been equal. In essence, while a lot of women have a few babies, a few men make a lot of babies. Anthropologists believe this is why they found double the number of female ancestors than male when analysing hundreds of genomes around the world. Social psychologist Roy F. Baumeister described it as the 'single most underappreciated fact about gender'. To get that kind of difference, he explained, it meant that in all of human history, perhaps 80 per cent of women but only 40 per cent of men had reproduced.

Around five thousand years ago, for every seventeen women that produced offspring, only one man did the same. In more recent times it has been five women for every man. Super sperm donors seem to be continuing that trend, while skewing the numbers even further. It has never been easier to purchase donor sperm online and more people than ever are actively seeking it out. In the western world, it is more socially acceptable for same-sex couples and single women to raise a family, but it seems that many are inadvertently using the same sperm donors.

In 2023, the mother of one of Jonathan Jacob Meijer's biological children – 'the man with 1000 kids' – took him to court. It was the first case of its kind and after hearing the evidence the judge ordered Meijer to stop donating, or face a €100,000 fine each time he did. Any clinics still holding his sperm were ordered to destroy it. Meijer described it as a 'legal castration' and according to the filmmakers it was the first time a court had successfully restricted a male's bodily autonomy. I paused the TV and rewound it. I couldn't believe what I was hearing. Not a day goes by when the bodily autonomy of a woman isn't involved in a legal battle or the subject of heated debate in the news. Abortion, rape, contraception, breastfeeding, fertility treatment. Nearly 50 per cent of women worldwide lack bodily autonomy because of power disparity and the threat of coercion or violence in their country. Some face prison or even death for choosing what to do with their own bodies, and yet here was the first case of a man being ordered to do the same. I was astonished.

We live in an age obsessed with true crime television shows. It's one of the reasons why I've stayed steadily employed over the last ten years. Interestingly, women make up the majority of the audience, being twice as likely as men to consume such content. Knowledge is power, perhaps. Face your fears in the comfort of your own home.

While filming crime documentaries, I never felt the need to watch them at home; I lived inside them, having a front-row seat to the action at work. I was in the passenger seat of police cars as they sped at ninety miles an hour down the motorway for an armed drugs raid. I was on the shoulders of paramedics as they responded to a triple stabbing or a five-car pile up. I was at crime scenes within minutes of the crime, tiptoeing around knives and needles, traipsing in fresh blood. I have cried with families whose child or brother was murdered. I have seen dead bodies and videos of child abuse; things we blur out for TV audiences. I have witnessed depravity up close, undiluted and unsanitised. I have been a shadow and a second skin to the trauma and the terror. No wonder I didn't seek it out in my spare time.

The sobering truth is that I have also been a part of the media wheel that uses the jeopardy of people's real lives as fodder for entertainment. When I began my career I was encouraged to see the work as educational and informative. I remember being told that recruitment rates for the ambulance service improved when our programmes broadcast and that we were offering the public a more human side to law enforcement. Personally, I know I've always done my best to look after the people I've filmed and have not pressured anyone into taking part in a TV programme, but at times it has still felt like an ethically dubious space in which to earn a living. It's something I've struggled with over the years.

Many of the adult children in the sperm donor films have described themselves as 'guinea pigs' or 'medical experiments', and I can't help but wonder what the next generation will think when they, and their peers, inevitably come to watch the TV programmes about how they were conceived. Learning that your parents fought a legal battle to convict your biological father while the whole world watched – in between episodes of their favourite sitcom – will be a lot to digest psychologically. We need to support these people as they grow older and come to terms with where they came from.

As a viewer, I was glad to see that most of the adult children appeared to be well-adjusted and remarkably accepting of the sinister circumstances of their conception. Perhaps their parents talking openly about it has served as an antidote to shame. Many even have a sense of humour about it all. What else is left to do but laugh when your own existence is an ethical minefield worthy of a Netflix true crime series?

In one of the films, in a strange twist of fate, one doctor-conceived woman explains that her dad – the man who raised her – is a funeral attendant. When the doctor – her biological father – died in 2017, it happened to be her dad who placed him in the coffin and buried him.

Time

Definition

1. A measurable period of duration
2. Events which succeed one another
3. An opportune or suitable moment

'You have a lovely garden,' I said, peering through the window. 'Thank you. We had a brilliant gardener, but unfortunately he killed himself,' John replied, then paused. 'Not because of the garden.'

I liked John already. I'd been in his house only a few minutes and his dark sense of humour was already twinkling. The story of his gardener reminded me of one my dad tells, about the man who built our fireplace, who also, sadly, took his own life. Again, not because of the fireplace.

I wanted to meet John Webster because he had been one of the doctors who delivered the world's first IVF baby – Louise Brown, on 25 July 1978 – and probably the only other person still alive who was in the room that night. Seven years after Louise was born, John and one of his colleagues, Simon Fishel, set up an IVF clinic in Nottinghamshire, the first of its kind in the Midlands. It was there that my parents became his patients.

John was tall, with thick white hair, large ears and a gracious smile. His skin was smooth and bright. I couldn't believe he was in his late eighties – he looked at least fifteen years younger. Some people seem to defy time, I thought.

It felt fitting that John shared his name with a Jacobean playwright, John Webster, a peer of Shakespeare. As an English and Drama graduate, I had spent many hours of my teens and twenties studying sixteenth-century plays. I like to think of this John as a kind of playwright too, of my life and many others. He may not have written the books, but he bound them together.

John introduced me to his wife Barbara then invited me into the living room, where he sat in an armchair and I perched on the sofa opposite. On the mantelpiece were two small clocks, ticking loudly, like heartbeats.

I asked if he minded me recording the audio of our interview.

'Of course,' he replied, in his Lancashire accent. I placed my phone on the coffee table in front of him. As I sank back into the sofa, I asked him to start from the very beginning.

'My dad was a butcher,' he said, 'but I always wanted to do medicine. I qualified in 1960 in Liverpool and needed some experience in obstetrics and gynaecology, but there wasn't a job at the hospital where I was working. A friend of mine said, oh I work for a guy called Patrick Steptoe, I'll give him a call. He was quite an amazing man, Steptoe. He pioneered laparoscopy and of course, that led to keyhole surgery becoming such an important part of medicine, which has probably been of more value to mankind than IVF.'

It was an interesting observation from a man whose entire career had revolved around IVF. It made me think about what 'value' means in the medical world. Is it the number of patients you treat or how much you improve their quality of life? Is it about delaying death or creating life?

'It was hard work,' John continued, 'because there was all this criticism, which Bob and Patrick batted away.'

'Were you ever affected by the criticism?' I asked.

'I was shielded from it, really. Patrick and Bob took all the flak. No, I had no concerns about it at all. I thought it was essential.

Because infertility had been treated very ineffectively for years and years. I thought it was going to be an essential part of medicine.'

I nodded, warmed by his faith that they were doing something meaningful.

'It was a tremendous undertaking, and it was just a sideline for us,' John said. 'We did egg collections early in the morning, before we started our NHS work, or at lunchtime, and embryo transfers at night.' Naively, I had not realised that IVF had not been their full-time job; they were doing it in their spare time, sacrificing lunch breaks and time with their families.

'We didn't have control of ovulation like we do now and the first pregnancy occurred in a lady, but she had an ectopic pregnancy. And then there were two or three other pregnancies that ended in miscarriage.'

The journey to making the world's first IVF baby was anything but straightforward. After a decade of trying and failing to achieve a full-term pregnancy, the wider scientific community had their doubts.

'Then, of course, in July 1978, Louise Brown came on the scene.'

'Tell me about that day,' I said.

'It was a Tuesday night and Patrick said meet me in the theatre at ten o'clock, we're going to do the Caesarean section. Only the essential staff knew, the porters weren't there,' said John, 'so Patrick and myself went down to the private block to pick up Lesley [Brown]. We walked along this long corridor and he suddenly said to me, I bet they wish they had me now.' John paused. 'Patrick Steptoe's one problem was not getting a job at St George's Hospital in London when he qualified. He used to bring it up every so often, this job at George's, which he thought he was absolutely suited to. And he never got it, so he came up to Oldham. And now here he was, the man who was going to deliver the world's first test-tube baby.'

Even those who achieve worldwide acclaim have their deeply

felt moments of rejection. After being overlooked for the job in London, Steptoe had been forced to pivot on to another path and patch, reluctantly relocating his family to the outskirts of Manchester where he set up a small practice. It seemed to me that Steptoe and Edwards had been spurred on as much by their critics as by their supporters, driven by the human need to prove themselves in the eyes of those who did not believe in them.

'Afterwards, Bob and Jeannie [Purdy] came over to the house I was renting from the hospital, and we had cheese on toast and a cup of tea,' said John. 'What a way to celebrate!'

'A very British way to celebrate,' I laughed.

The story of the miracle baby made the front pages of newspapers all around the world. Finally there existed a way for infertile couples to have children of their own. But instead of being offered jobs and shiny new laboratories to extend their work to more people, Edwards, Steptoe and Purdy found themselves abandoned. The British Medical Research Council continued to refuse them funding and the newspaper that had offered to finance their next venture abruptly bailed on them because the new owner's wife opposed IVF.

The small team spent two years raising money and trying to find a suitable place to open a private clinic. One day Purdy stumbled across a secluded four-hundred-year-old manor house in the Cambridgeshire countryside. It wasn't a hospital, but it was a decent size, so they took a gamble and renovated it. In September 1980 the world's first dedicated IVF clinic opened, aptly named Bourn Hall.

'There was no razzmatazz,' John said. 'We just opened up and waited for people to come.' In those days there was no internet and doctors were not allowed to advertise. With no coverage, there were no queues of patients lining up.

After a few months it looked like the clinic might have to shut down. At Oldham they'd had four thousand people on the waiting list so John sought out the files from Patrick Steptoe's secretary and began phoning round.

'Initially I couldn't get hold of anybody,' he said, 'and then I realised, no kids, they're probably both at work in the daytime. So I started phoning at night, and that's when I started getting through. And I did that night after night.' From there word of mouth helped, because a lot of the patients knew one another, having been at the clinic at the same time and staying in contact. 'Then it just took off.'

As different kinds of patients and scenarios arose, John and his colleagues realised they needed to know the parameters that they could work within and ideally some legislation from the government. 'I don't think any of us knew how big it was going to be,' John said, 'but we needed some guidance, some rules setting down, and about twelve of us met at a hotel in London to discuss how we should try and get a sort of organisation together, which led to the HFEA being established.'

The Human Fertilisation and Embryology Authority was formed in 1991, thirteen years after the first IVF baby and the same year I was born. It was the first regulatory body of assisted reproduction treatment in the world and provided a blueprint for many other countries going forward.

Sandra and John Coxon met John Webster in 1985. He was their main point of contact at the fertility clinic, answering questions and performing the egg collections and embryo transfers. They trusted him, and I could see why. He was easy to talk to, and despite our fifty-five-year age gap and having only just met, I felt like I could talk to him about anything and it would be met with empathy and understanding.

I wanted to know what it was like for my parents back then. What stigma was there for people seeking fertility treatment in the 1980s and 1990s?

'The UK was a bit more religious back then, and people would ask how we got the soul into the embryo and that sort of thing. I don't think some people really understood what was going on. And the press had a lot to answer for. Whenever there was an article on IVF they always showed a picture of a test tube with a little baby trying to crawl out of it, which wasn't very nice.'

John's landline phone started ringing and he excused himself to go and answer it.

'Hello, Betty, how are you?' I overheard. 'Oh, well, listen, Betty, I've got a lady here, as a result of IVF, who I'm just doing an interview with. So I'll let her know about you. Oh, we're talking about the history of it. Yeah. How old is James now, by the way? Forty-one. Okay, I'll call you back.'

John returned to the living room, smiling.

'That was a lady called Betty, from Scotland. Her son is forty-one now. He was IVF too.'

'Oh, wow. He must have been a really early one then?'

'Fairly early, yeah.'

'Because Louise will be forty-six this year.'

'Gosh. I'll have to hang on another four years then, for when she turns fifty,' John said, and we both laughed, uneasily.

I asked what kind of response he got from the families after he'd helped them have children.

'They were always grateful, very grateful,' he replied, then looked away. 'They weren't the problem though, it was supporting the ones who didn't get pregnant. When I was counselling people, I told them it's a two out of three chance of it failing every time.'

'And it still is, isn't it?'

'It's not got a whole lot better, no. I knew one woman, it caused her a lot of heartache. She committed suicide because she couldn't get pregnant.'

My heart sank. I was reminded of Doris Del Zio and the depression she had experienced when her IVF procedure ended badly. Fifty years later and again the United States was being confronted with a similarly poignant story. 'I don't know if you've read about the news in America,' I said. 'About a patient who accidentally dropped some embryos on the floor?'

'No,' he said. 'I try to stay out of it now.'

We were meeting three months after a supreme court in Alabama had ruled that embryos were 'extrauterine children', resulting in the immediate closure of several IVF clinics in the state. The court decision had come about after an incident in December 2020 in which a patient of a fertility clinic had wandered into a cryogenic storage unit and picked up a container of frozen embryos. She freeze-burned her hand and accidentally dropped the embryos on the floor, destroying them. The three different couples to whom they belonged went on to sue the clinic for wrongful death of a minor, which a court eventually rejected because it considered embryos to be property, not people, when they exist outside of a womb. The couples appealed their case to the state supreme court, which ruled in their favour, deciding that the frozen embryos should be considered their 'children', sending shockwaves through the country.

'So they're essentially saying that those children have been murdered,' I explained, 'and the IVF clinics said, well we can't practise IVF safely in the eyes of the law now because there will be embryos that are destroyed.'

'There will always be accidents,' John said.

'Accidents, or, if they don't use all the embryos and end up discarding some because they're of poor quality or they already have enough children, are they committing murder?' I took a pause for breath. 'And what about freezing embryos, where do they stand legally?' I asked, as if John might have the answers to these decades-old philosophical questions.

'Mmm,' he mumbled. 'Well, I mean, the Americans are so conscious of litigation, aren't they?'

A few weeks after the supreme court ruling, the state passed a law protecting IVF clinics from liability in the case of damaged or destroyed embryos, allowing fertility clinic staff to resume their work. But it did not address the legal status of embryos or fertilised eggs. The question being, at what point in time does a clump of cells become a legal 'person'?

Some argue that embryos are capable of life but do not yet consist of life, while others believe that life begins at the moment of conception, when sperm and egg merge. In the UK and Europe, a foetus does not have rights of its own until it is born and exists separately from the mother, though legally it is not 'nothing' and is considered differently, for example, to a limb.

In the US, in the years since the Supreme Court rescinded the constitutional right to abortion, the 'fetal personhood' movement has been gathering pace, seeking to secure more rights, privileges and immunities to 'unborn children', including embryos created during IVF.

'So they're having a bit of a conundrum in America at the moment about what it means,' I said. 'Forty-five years after Louise Brown, it's a very interesting time again.'

'It's an interesting time to be out of it,' said John, with a smirk. While I was getting my head into these debates for the first time, I realised it was familiar, and probably tedious, territory for John. He had already mentioned that he didn't have a mobile phone because he'd 'had enough phone calls in the past', and getting hold of him hadn't been easy; I had to write a letter and have it delivered by someone who knew where he lived.

These days, he said, he preferred to live a quiet life, playing golf three times a week and spending time with his three sons and five granddaughters.

'I had a heart attack last year. I was playing golf and one of my pals took me to hospital. I ended up having two stents, but when they were putting the second stent in, the blood vessel burst and my heart stopped for half an hour.'

'Oh gosh,' I said.

'So they resuscitated me and I was in hospital for two months. And since then my memory's not so good.'

'You've done absolutely brilliantly, your memory is amazing,' I said. I asked if there was anything else he wanted people to know.

'Well, when it comes down to it,' he said, 'it's not how babies are conceived, it's how you bring them up.'

In my late twenties, my friends and I used to fantasise about having children at the same time. We daydreamed about coffee dates and park strolls with our prams, the names we liked, our kids being best friends. In the six years since, I have watched many of their bodies change and grow, expand and compress. Inhale and exhale; as easy as breathing. Some of them have given birth two or three times over. And I look on from the shoreline, waiting for my time. Years have passed. Their babies have grown into toddlers and children, losing their first teeth and bringing home certificates from school. I love being 'Auntie Bex', always prepared with a sticker book, crayons and a hand to hold, but every milestone in their lives feels like a splinter in mine.

'It'll be the right time for you, when it happens,' Mum tells me, and I try my best to believe her.

As I listen back to the audio recording of my interview with John, all I can hear are the clocks on his mantelpiece ticking away; almost upstaging us. The rhythmic sound underpins our conversation so literally I can't help but wince at how glaring the metaphor is. As John's heart ticks on, I hope he will live to see his first IVF baby turn fifty in a few years. In the meantime I dream of growing a second heart myself one day. I cannot think of a sound more beautiful than a heartbeat ticking on a sonogram.

For both of us, time is running out.

*

A few years ago when my siblings and I arrived home for the Christmas holidays, we sat around the kitchen table chatting and drinking together.

'Get out the tape measure again,' Mum said to Dad. He stood up and walked out of the room. I assumed he was going to start measuring a table leg or oak beam and get our opinions on a new renovation project or something, but when he came back he pulled the tape measure out to a hundred inches and laid it across the table. He pointed his finger around two-thirds along.

'This is where I am,' he said, then slowly moved his finger along the line, from seventy back to zero. 'Look at the amount of life I've already lived.'

He asked us all to point to our age on the tape measure.

'Look at how much life you've lived and how long you've got left. And you're lucky if you live to ninety or a hundred.' We nodded and looked at each other. He put the tape measure away, picked up his glass of wine and we continued as if nothing had happened.

It was a rather Dickensian way to get us into the Christmas spirit, but the blunt reality is that the older we are when we have our children, the less time we get to spend with them. This truth stalks me, not only when it comes to my own children but with my parents too. They are in their mid-seventies now; they had to wait for IVF to be invented before they could have children, and they were just in time. When I was born, Mum was thirty-nine and Dad was forty. The thought of them not being around to spend time with my children is one that chokes me so tightly that I am barely able to write it down. I did not meet either of my grandfathers – they both died before I was born. I have very few memories of my grandmothers who both died while I was young. I cannot conceive of this for my own children, I do not want to.

One of the symptoms of infertility is time. We are all born

infertile and most of us die infertile. In our finite reproductive years, infertility is defined as a heterosexual couple being unable to get pregnant after twelve months or more of regular unprotected sex. For single women or lesbian couples it is not conceiving after six rounds of donor insemination. For gay men the barriers to conceiving children are immense; often even more costly and time-consuming. When they discover that they need fertility treatment, many people are racing against the clock, trying not to let time outpace their chances. Some people are fertile at a time when they, or their partner, do not yet feel ready for children, only to find that when the 'right' time comes along, the biological fact of ageing has already begun to work against them.

In 2010, Robert Edwards was awarded the Nobel Prize for developing IVF, but it came too late. In the three decades since his team's scientific breakthrough, Jean Purdy and Patrick Steptoe had died, and Edwards was too unwell to attend the ceremony. He had vascular dementia and those closest to him believe that by then he wasn't even able to understand that he'd received the award. He died three years later.

It is a tragedy that we did not recognise Steptoe, Purdy and Edwards in time, but there is comfort in knowing that their legacy lives on through the twelve million people, including me, alive today because of them. And, if we're lucky, the millions more children and grandchildren that will follow.

Space

Definition

1. The area beyond the Earth's atmosphere
2. A period of time
3. The distance between us

My body was strapped to a man I'd only just met. My sister-in-law, Gina, was grinning. I was glad she was there, I felt safer. Then she disappeared and I panicked. A few seconds later, the man and I were shuffling our bums forward and we jumped out of the plane too.

Suddenly we were free-falling. Terminal velocity, 120 miles per hour. Time feels slower up there, when you're diving from the sky, dicing with life. There was no resistance, just our bodies plummeting through empty space. I saw Gina again, in front, giving me a double thumbs up.

Then Mum jumped out of the plane, and, later, the rest of my family did too. In August 2020 – for Mum's sixty-ninth birthday – we were doing a family skydive. Tim and Gina had set it up, being regular skydivers. For the rest of us it was a once-in-a-lifetime experience, but for them it was just a normal weekend.

My older brother, Tim, had fallen for skydiving in his early twenties after doing a tandem dive while on holiday in New Zealand. Two years later, he met Gina. Eventually she got bored of watching him go skydiving with his friends all the time and decided to have a go herself. Since then they've bought matching jumpsuits and dived out of hundreds of planes together around the world, even completing extra qualifications allowing them to jump in group formations. The photographs of these formations are stunning. Four people holding hands and seated as if at a table, but upside down. They look like gods, creating their own celestial architecture in the sky, the clouds at their feet, the earth above them. With the sunrise squinting in the corner, the earth below looks slightly spherical. I find the images very moving, perhaps because their lives are literally in the balance, but also because it's a view of the world so few of us get to see.

Some years after her first skydive, Gina got a job as a professional 'wing walker'. One day she was an estate agent and the next she was performing acrobatics on top of a biplane. At two thousand feet she would climb out of the cockpit on to the top wing, attach herself to a harness and bend her body into impressive shapes against the full force of the wind. These James Bond-style stunts were even more impressive when the plane was doing loop-the-loops, flying upside down or brushing past another plane so closely that the two wing walkers could hold hands, and sometimes they did. For two years Gina toured the world like this – from France to China – with the Breitling Wingwalkers, entertaining crowds at airshows. Afterwards children would line up for photos with her, inspired to fly.

On the day of our family skydive, Gina was in the very early stages of pregnancy, though she didn't know it yet. A tiny embryo had implanted into her womb; the youngest skydiver in the world.

When we were children, our playroom was space-themed. The wallpaper was adorned with suns and moons and the ceiling was tacked with glow-in-the-dark stars that lit up at night. We had rocket-shaped lava lamps and posters of Neil Armstrong in his NASA spacesuit. Our trips to Leicester Space Centre and the Planetarium in London were my favourite days out. When I learned about other galaxies and black holes, it gave me a profound and piercing sense of how insignificant I was in relation to the universe.

When IVF pioneers Robert Edwards and Jean Purdy saw four developing embryos for the first time it gave them the same feeling; of being humbled and dwarfed by nature. It was the moment, Edwards said, 'when everything became possible'. Later that evening, as Edwards walked to his car, intoxicated by his unexpected breakthrough, he wrote: 'I looked up at all the stars, the moon, the night sky over Oldham, and considered the equally amazing sights I had just seen under my microscope.'

In the 1960s, while some scientists were looking up at the moon, others were looking down a lens into a different kind of solar system: one of spermatozoa, ova, zygotes and blastocysts. Not the names of aliens or asteroids but the earliest moments of conception, never witnessed before. As we began to explore the vastness of space, we were also examining the minutiae of life. While astronomers pondered life on other planets, embryologists wondered whether we could create life from scratch ourselves. President Kennedy wanted to land on the moon before the decade was over. 'Whether it will become a force for good or ill depends on man,' he said, while ethicists were having the same debate about growing humans in the laboratory.

'To be the first ... to engage single-handed in an unprecedented duel with nature – could anyone dream of anything greater than that?' Those were the words of twenty-seven-year-old Yuri Gagarin, the Soviet cosmonaut, before he boarded the rocket that would propel him into orbit and make him the first human in space. But the same words could have been describing IVF; both were dabbling with the divine, both were an unprecedented duel with nature.

Six foot. Blonde hair. Blue eyes. Medical student. This was the only information the clinic gave my parents about the sperm donor. It seems like every sperm donor at the time was some sort of Aryan scientist. Smart, fair, tall. But, like dating profiles, it's hard to believe. Did they just tell the parents what they wanted to hear? In a culture of anonymity, did they even keep track of which sperm donors were used for which family? In any case, these on-paper facts don't tell us anything about someone's personality; their sense of humour, their hobbies, their music taste, the way they walk or talk or how generous they are. It is a mystery, a gamble. A marble cake of DNA, a swirling galaxy of genetics.

Tim has brown hair, green eyes and is five foot ten. He's the only one in our family with a cleft chin. He is a good listener and always looks like he's about to laugh. He completed his Master's degree in quantum physics, studying black holes, and turned down a PhD. Electrodynamics, localised surface plasmon, nanoparticles; he uses words I don't understand, but for all his nerdiness he is also quite cool. He goes to drum and bass raves and gets a backstage pass to Glastonbury every year. He makes his own fireworks, most famously the 'human Catherine wheel' that rivets us all every Bonfire Night. Attaching steel wool to the end of two thick wires, he douses them in paraffin and sets them on fire. Then he spins them – one in each hand, as fast as he can – creating a spectacular ring of flying sparks around him. A whole-body halo.

Bonfire Night is one of the few times we gather annually as a family and November 2022 was no different. We were all wrapped up warm and sitting outside on plastic chairs in my parents' garden around a fire pit. I was mesmerised by the flames rioting above; smoke rising and disappearing into the night sky. Blocks of wood morphing from something into nothing. Tim's eighteen-month-old daughter, Ava, was sitting on his lap while the rest of us caught up on the previous months; holidays, house moves, work.

'Guess where Tim's next project will be based?' Gina asked.

My brother designed internet data centres for a living and so far all of his projects had been based in rural towns near the M25.

'Scotland?' I answered.

'Further away,' Gina replied.

I tried to think of countries with vast amounts of space, large enough to build warehouses.

'Iceland?'

'Nope. Further.'

'New Zealand?'

'No, further.'

I was stumped.

'Hawaii?'

'Even further,' she replied.

Oh.

'Mars?'

Gina laughed.

'No, not that far.'

'The moon!'

'Yes.'

Everyone gasped. Tim announced he was working on a project that would put a data centre on the moon. Led by a company called Lonestar and launched by SpaceX, it would be the first in history to provide a commercial service from the lunar surface. The data, he explained, would be safeguarded from the unpredictability of the Earth's elements: fire, floods, war. If the world combusted, there would be something of modern technology and humanity left. The moon – void of weather or atmosphere, and a natural satellite of our planet – provided an ideal location to store such crucial information.

Since he was a small child, Tim has been taking things apart and putting them back together again; learning how they work, glimpsing into their guts, analysing their anatomy. Toys, computers, robots, cars. He once bought a disused ambulance and turned it into a campervan like it was no big deal. In his early twenties he constructed a bitcoin-mining supercomputer that not only *made* him money but ran so hot that it doubled as a heater for his home, *saving* him money.

Tim told us he would be helping establish the ground satellite link in the UK, just a small role, but important nevertheless. I felt so proud of him; he was making history.

Mum was in the house preparing food, but I knew she'd want to be part of the conversation. I skipped inside to tell her.

'Oh my god, I've got tingles,' she said, covering the sausages in foil. 'Can he take me with him?'

I laughed. 'But would you really want to go into space?'

'I've always wanted to go.'

'Why?'

'I want to see this,' she said, searching for a picture on her phone. She showed me the photograph, called *Earthrise*, taken by astronaut Bill Anders in 1968, when she was seventeen. Half in shadow, the Earth appears fluorescent against the black night sky, rising above the lunar landscape. The crew were supposed to be taking photos of the moon, but as Anders looked out the tiny window of the spacecraft he 'suddenly saw this object called Earth'. It was, he said, 'the only colour in the universe'.

The astronaut scrambled for his camera, set the focus to infinity and started shooting. Amid the Cold War, the Vietnam War and the recent assassinations of Martin Luther King Jr and the Kennedy brothers, the photograph, of Earth as a whole, was described as a moment for global reflection and unity.

Later that day, on Christmas Eve 1968, the Apollo 8 mission broadcast live from their lunar orbit to millions of people around the world. Against grainy images of the moon, Anders and his crewmates read from the book of Genesis:

'In the beginning, God created the heavens and the Earth. And the Earth was without form, and void; and darkness was upon the face of the deep. And the Spirit of God moved upon the face of the waters. And God said, let there be light.'

The irony of their chosen reading – so at odds with the scientific understanding of how the Earth came to be – was not lost on some viewers. In fact, Anders later admitted his experience in space 'really undercut' his religious beliefs. Previously a devout Catholic, he lost his faith as a result of his spaceflight.

For seventeen-year-old Sandra, *Earthrise* sparked something. For my mother, now in her seventh decade, I wanted to know why. What was it about seeing the Earth like this that she craved?

'I like the idea of separation from the world,' she said, 'but also knowing I'd come back.'

In January 1986, thirty-four-year-old Sandra was sitting in a hospital bed glued to the television. Christa McAuliffe was about to become the first civilian in space and Sandra was fizzing with envy. A high school teacher from New Hampshire and mother of two, McAuliffe had beaten eleven thousand other teachers to win a seat on the Space Shuttle Challenger mission. After six months of training, the shuttle launched on 28 January, the same day Sandra was undergoing her first IVF embryo transfer.

'Good afternoon, Mrs Coxon,' Dr John Webster said, as he entered the room.

But Mum did not take her eyes off the screen.

'The Challenger has just blown up,' she said.

'What?'

'The Challenger Space Shuttle has just blown up.'

Dr Webster had been intending to tell Sandra how many embryos they'd managed to fertilise from the eggs they'd collected from her ovaries days before. But instead they were both staring at the television in disbelief.

After months of exciting build-up the world had counted down as the shuttle lifted off. There had been seventy-three seconds of cheering from the crowd. Elation, awe, possibility. Then, silence from mission control. A fireball ripping through the indigo sky. Pearl-coloured smoke catapulting in two directions, like a wishbone. There was no more rocket. Where had it gone?

In the footage a chorus of cheers and screams can be heard from the crowd, everyone looking at each other for answers but no one having any. Debris rains from the sky as the children Christa taught watch on in horror from the launch site. Their teacher had just been blown up in front of them. Millions more children were watching from their school classrooms. The live streaming cameras continue to roll on the faces of Christa's parents as they realise, in real time, what everyone hopes in their bones not to be true. But everyone knew; an explosion like that could leave no survivors. How could this have happened? There was no explanation, just silence and an inconceivable loss.

And still, Mum wants to go into space.

'They found some wreckage in Florida this week, did you see?' I asked, gathering a selection of sauces from the fridge.

'Yeah, it gave me shivers,' she replied.

'The first time in twenty-five years that they've recovered any of it.'

'I'll never forget watching it live.'

Back in her hospital bed, Sandra knew her chances of conceiving were low: just 7 per cent. After artificially stimulating her ovaries with medication the previous week, the fertility team had managed to collect just two eggs. Of those, one had developed into a good-quality embryo, ready to be transferred into her womb that afternoon.

As the embryo nestled into its new home, Sandra was told to rest. Don't even lift a kettle for the next two weeks, they said. All she needed to do was let her body protect it. A fortnight later, after nine years of trying, Sandra and John had their first ever positive pregnancy test.

But then something else blew up. Chernobyl. This time news reporters warned of a giant toxic cloud expanding over Europe, encroaching on our airspace. Nuclear radiation causing catastrophic contamination. Cancer. Cataracts. Foetal deformities. Radioactive milk. The worst nuclear disaster in history. How could this have happened? Terrified of the noxious fumes poisoning the fragile life she had spent so many years trying to create, Sandra shut the windows and didn't leave the house for six weeks.

I headed back outside, placed the sauces and cutlery on the table and sat back down next to Tim.

'Will you get to go to the moon?' I asked.

'No,' he laughed. 'But I suppose there is a possibility, if something needs fixing.'

I looked up at the bright, full moon and the fire pit smoke dancing around it.

'I would trust you to fix anything,' I said. 'You might have to take Mum with you, though.'

Tissue

Definition

1. A group of connected cells that have the same function
2. A piece of soft absorbent paper

A few days ago I sneezed while peeing and it felt like my bladder had ripped in half. Sometimes I get a gut feeling – not a useful sense of intuition, I can actually *feel* my gut and it's like pushing a cactus through my colon. Occasionally I have to stop myself from yelping on the toilet because the pain is unbearable. Then it passes, I take some tissue, flush and carry on with my day. It's so normal now that I don't mention it to anyone. What could they do anyway? I wish the stabs of my splintered intestines were the worst part about living with endometriosis, but it's actually the symptom I find the most easy to ignore.

For the last few years I have lived in an on/off state of what I call 'half-sickness'. Not ill enough to stay in bed but not well enough to function properly. If you've ever had the flu – when you feel exhausted and every bone in your body aches – it is something like that, yet for me it happens almost weekly.

I know my body is only trying its best. My immune system thinks I'm being attacked and is retaliating, but my body is fighting a war it will never win. It's not a sword fight with an invading enemy; I'm being infiltrated from the inside, cyber-hacked by my own employees. It requires different weapons, yet my body throws flamethrowers and grenades anyway.

Contrary to popular belief, endometriosis is not a 'menstrual' condition. It doesn't just cause 'bad periods' and preventing periods does not stop the symptoms, nor does it only affect the reproductive organs. It is a chronic, inflammatory, systemic condition that affects the whole body. I wish more people knew this.

The reason my body is in a regular state of stress is because there is rogue tissue in parts of my body where there shouldn't be. This tissue skulks in the nooks of my abdomen, sticking to the pelvic walls and burrowing into organs. It is similar to the womb-lining – the endometrium – but not quite the same. It responds to the hormones of the menstrual cycle, often exacerbating pain at certain times of the month, but that's not the full story. Once the tissue has embedded itself, it can behave in unpredictable ways. While normal tissue is a soft pink, endometriosis can be red, blue, white, black or yellow. Over time organs become dotted by 'gunshot' lesions; small black cysts that look like fish roe.

Endometriosis is usually found within the pelvic cavity – on the ovaries, fallopian tubes, bladder, bowels and uterus – but in rare cases it has been found as far afield as the diaphragm, lungs and brain. The tissue is metastatic; invading and thriving on multiple organs, damaging them on the surface and sometimes deeper. In many ways it behaves like a cancer that doesn't kill you.

For some people the tissue develops into large sticky adhesions like chewing gum, fusing organs together. Lesions can even develop their own nerve and hormone supply. But no matter how hard the body tries to eject the cells or repair the organs, it cannot get rid of the unwanted tissue and thus the body becomes chronically inflamed.

Because endometriosis has invaded my bladder and bowels, when I use the toilet my inner tubing often feels bruised, like a needle has been pushed through the plumbing of my pelvis. Rusty drains, corroding pipework. Some days it feels like a bottle of hot chilli sauce has been poured into my fuel tank, coating my gut, varnishing my bones. I picture a tattoo on a biker's bicep but rather than a flaming heart, it's a flaming womb. I've always been ambitious, but it gives a new meaning to the phrase 'fire in your belly'. For four days a month I bleed like a beer keg burst open with a knife.

If I talk in 'men's' terms, might they be more receptive to these female experiences? I wonder. Might they not turn away from the language of human anatomy so readily, thinking it irrelevant or worse, hysterical? The least we can all do is listen, and if we dare to demand more? Put as much funding into research and treatment for endometriosis as we do for medical issues that commonly affect men. As it stands there is five times more funded research into erectile dysfunction – a condition that affects 19 per cent of men – than into premenstrual syndrome, which affects 90 per cent of women.

The only definitive way to diagnose endometriosis is through keyhole surgery. Since surgery is invasive and waiting lists are often long, experts believe it is vastly underdiagnosed. For others it is misdiagnosed – as irritable bowel syndrome or mental illness – or ignored by health professionals as a normal part of being female. Bad periods, cramps, PMS; no big deal, pop a painkiller, stop making a fuss. In the UK it takes an average of eight years to get a diagnosis. Meanwhile the disease progresses.

When endometriosis is diagnosed by laparoscopy, the surgery is more complex than other abdominal surgery because it usually involves pelvic sidewalls and multiple organs – including the fragile ovaries – so it cannot be performed by a regular gynaecologist. The possible side effects of surgery are sobering: reduced ovarian reserve, scar tissue, organ damage. And even then surgery is not a cure; endometriosis often comes back. Recurrence rates after surgery are 20 per cent within two years and 50 per cent within five years.

Six years on from my surgery, I know mine has grown back

with more fervour, I can feel it. Every few days the symptoms inch back into my life like a vine wrapping around a tree trunk, strangling my organs. Inflammation bubbles through my veins like lava, ready to erupt at any time. When my tabby cat affectionately kneads my belly with his paws, it feels like he's using knuckle dusters. The pain can be devious, the way it prowls – at first from a safe distance, captive and under control one week, then a sudden frenzy of tugging and snarling the next. Fight or flight? What to do when your body is the battlefield and the war is between your own fibres?

Endometriosis affects one in ten women of reproductive age and yet many people haven't heard of it. While most women are diagnosed in their twenties or thirties, endometriosis has also been found in prepubescent girls, elderly women and female foetuses. There have also been a few reports of endometriosis in cis men, however these were mostly men being given high doses of oestrogen for the treatment of prostate cancer in the 1950s and 1960s, which is no longer prescribed. To put it into context, while the condition affects around two hundred million girls and women worldwide, there have been less than twenty documented cases in boys or men. If there were more cases in men, I've no doubt there would be more of a rush to find a cure.

We don't know why endometriosis develops in some women and not others, though there is often a strong genetic component. Women with a mother or sister with endometriosis, like me, face a seven-fold increased risk of having it themselves. But for an illness that is as common as diabetes or asthma, we know very little about it. Current treatments remain rudimentary, ineffective and come with side effects like preventing ovulation and temporary or permanent menopause. While we spend billions on diabetes and asthma every year, it feels like a great injustice that funding for endometriosis research continues to operate on a shoestring.

Some days I am okay; not a twinge. My anatomy is mine again and the day can proceed as I intend. Other days I wake up with a body made of timber. Rebecca, the wooden girl, not quite a real one. On these days it takes great effort to concentrate on anything, brain fog being another common symptom. Sleeping is not safe either as I'm awoken by my belly, burning and sore, with cramps refusing to be contained to waking hours. I toss and turn trying to get comfortable, but you can't crawl away from your own insides. I wake up scrambled, haunted by fatigue, wading through tar for the rest of the day. As pain dominates, hunger dissipates. I eat out of courtesy to my body and feel nothing. Chew, swallow, digest. Conditions like these take away many things from people, but how dare the simple pleasures of appetite and satiation be among them? These are the things they do not tell you in textbooks. These are the things difficult to describe when someone asks 'How are you?'

Over the years I have joined support groups and read books about the best diets for managing endometriosis. Among them they advise avoiding sugar, alcohol, dairy, soy, caffeine, processed food, certain fruits and vegetables, red meat and gluten. What, I wonder, is left? What small pleasures remain?

Interestingly, women diagnosed with endometriosis tend to have a lower body mass index than the average population. Researchers don't know why, but I wonder if it has something to do with our hunger being stalled by pain and bloating – the infamous 'endo belly' – and the restriction of different foods as we attempt to figure out what exacerbates our symptoms. In the meantime I hear of women who are overweight repeatedly being told by doctors that losing weight will improve their symptoms. I get the sense that most doctors have no idea what to say to endometriosis patients. How could they when medical science cannot even agree on what endometriosis is or how and why it develops? Many simply prescribe birth control pills or painkillers and send the patient on their way. This has not changed for the last forty years.

For me, some days painkillers help but other days they make no difference at all. Heat can take the edge off – a bath or hot water bottle – and in emergencies I use my small, portable TENS machine. Transcutaneous electrical nerve stimulation is a technology that emits electric pulses through small pads stuck to your skin. The surface-level vibrations distract your nerve signals from the internal pain and encourage the release of endorphins. It's usually recommended for women in labour.

My life has not always been this way. Once upon a time I was ignorant of the intricacies of dull aches and sore organs. I knew what a 'normal' cycle felt like so I know that this is not it. My job as a documentary director involves running around holding heavy cameras for hours at a time, filming on location for six-week stints and being woken up at all hours on-call. I have lived my life on the go, always moving, reacting and adapting to other people's schedules. My symptoms used to be manageable, if only just. That was, until I came off the pill. After over a decade of the progestogen-only pill quelling my symptoms, they have since surged. This is a common story. The tell-tale signs of endometriosis are often suppressed by the pill and many women are not confronted with them until they come off it.

The pill has always been controversial – heavy with a history of patriarchy, religion and unwanted side effects, and I support anyone who does not wish to ingest artificial hormones as a form of contraception – but for women with endometriosis, it feels like we have little choice. It is one of the only 'treatments' that currently exist, and yet it simply disguises the symptoms. There is no cure.

There are compounded challenges in having an illness that is invisible. Though my body's immune system is in overdrive and I often feel paralysed with fatigue, I tend to look fine. To an outsider, the only visible symptoms are a few stifled yawns, a glazed look in my eye and trousers with an elasticated waistband. I have learned how to feel pain and replace it with something else. I am skilled at the dark art of disassociating from my body. Detaching, disembodying. In the short term it helps me to cope, but if we press the mute button on our bodies we stop hearing everything: danger, hunger, butterflies. We become numb, and it's no way to live.

On my good days my family get the fun, happy version of me they know and love. I have energy, I have a sense of humour, I enjoy life. But then the symptoms return and I am engulfed by brutal pelvic pangs, aching bones and the panic of a future lassoed by misery. My cognitive monologue regresses to that of a toddler with the world's worst bellyache, furious at the unfairness of it all. My personality calcifies into someone resentful and mean. I am irritable. An inner loathing begins to unfurl between crevices of skin and bone. This is what your own tissue can do to you.

There are no bruises. No one can see the internal swelling, cramps or bleeding. I look the same as I always do. I imagine that many people with endo (and other chronic illnesses) worry that others judge them for having a low tolerance for pain, but I think the opposite is more likely to be true; we deal with pain so often that our threshold is high. We are far more likely to underplay our symptoms than overstate them. We become fluent in the language and accents of pain. There are plenty of women who say that their endometriosis pain is worse than their experience of childbirth.

In any case, I feel the need to quantify my relationship with pain. I returned to work the day after my keyhole surgery. I once had gum surgery without anaesthetic. I find smear tests relaxing. I once got second-degree burns on my thighs while filming a TV series and, after a stint in A&E, picked up my camera again a few hours later, bandages peeling off my bubbling skin. I have played sports at national level, routinely pushing my body as fast and far as it will go. I say these things not to impress anyone – my relationship with pain (and work) is probably not healthy – but because I want to reiterate that chronic pain is not a marker of how weak or resilient we are. We can be tough and still suffer.

I have a friend, Charlotte Henshaw, who is a Paralympian. We met on our county swim squad as teenagers. She competes in her sports – paracanoe and swimming – at the most elite level in the world. A few years ago, she was diagnosed with endometriosis and messaged me before her surgery to ask for advice. Since then she's talked openly in the media about her experiences with endo and I am always impressed by her eloquence and efforts in raising awareness. She has won gold, silver and bronze medals in five Paralympic Games and is a ten-time world champion, but on her bad days she says her symptoms are so debilitating that she can't do anything.

Welsh rugby player Ffion Lewis had her first endometriosis flare-up in the middle of a training session and found the pain to be so bad she thought she was dying. Australian swimmer Emily Seebohm has won three Olympic gold medals but says every day is a battle with endometriosis. Paralympic swimmer Monique Murphy said the pain of endometriosis was worse than losing her leg. In 2022 Leah Williamson led the England football team to victory in the European Championships final, but most people don't know that she nearly missed the game because of an endo flare-up.

These elite athletes have gruelling training schedules and test the boundaries of human physical capability for their job. But when your body is your instrument – your career and means of making a living – a life with endometriosis must feel even more complicated.

'At times it feels like this body I've been given is literally trying to attack me,' wrote American sprinter Brittany Brown on social media. 'But at the same time I love my body because it figures out a way to SHOW UP.'

Before winning bronze on her Olympic debut, Brown opened up about her endometriosis diagnosis, saying how she cried and vomited before one of the most important 200m races of her career. I am beyond impressed that these women manage to compete at all when their bodies rebel like this, never mind be among the best in the world. For black women, the hurdles to accessing support and treatment for endometriosis are even higher. When asked in an interview if she has dealt with medical racism, Brown replied:

> I think that when we talk about pain, Black women have always been told that we have a high pain threshold and we can handle it, so that dismissal that affects women's health issues in general is that much more extreme. I have connected with other Black women in the endo space who feel like they have to be that much more cautious. It starts with period pain, but this is also about concerns to do with childbirth and the possibility of surgery.

For decades endometriosis was considered a 'career woman's disease', and more specifically, a *white* career woman's disease. Unfortunately, today, black women are still less likely to receive a diagnosis, likely to wait longer for a diagnosis and more likely to receive poorer care when they are diagnosed.

In 2021, thirty-year-old Aubrion Rogers posted on an endometriosis support Facebook group asking for advice.

> I have been in pain daily for months. Today I went to urgent care and asked for an ultrasound. Found out that I have three fibroids, one cyst, one enlarged ovary and one large mass that is 11cm. At what point will my situation be considered an emergency? Is 11cm

not big enough?? They sent me home and told me to contact my doctor. I called him and can't get in until Monday. I'm so tired of this pain! I can barely work and I've been missing so many days. What can I do? Should I ask for a doctor's note for a couple of days, should I ask for pain meds, should I just keep going to work and struggle? Uhhhh.

Six months later, after three weeks of extreme pain, Rogers was admitted for emergency surgery to remove a large endometrioma that had caused her right ovary to burst. A few days later she died from complications of the surgery.

Had Rogers been taken seriously earlier, her condition would not have progressed so far, she would not have needed emergency surgery and her death might have been prevented.

In June 2024, thirty-eight-year-old radio host and DJ Jahmby Koikai died from complications of endometriosis, after years of campaigning for better healthcare for women in Kenya. It took her seventeen years to get her diagnosis, by which point her lung had collapsed from thoracic endometriosis. Koikai fundraised for specialist surgery in the US and was treated there for two years, but the delay in her treatment and previous botched surgeries meant it came too late.

I find these stories so appallingly sad. When I have spoken to doctors about my symptoms, I have always been taken seriously, but I know I am lucky. If Koikai and Rogers had been white women, I wonder if they'd have been offered better care and still be alive today.

Endometriosis is not new. According to Dr Camran Nezhat and his brothers, who wrote the medical paper 'Endometriosis: Ancient Disease, Ancient Treatments', endometriosis has been documented for thousands of years, under the guise of different names. Plato called it 'suffocation of the womb', while others described it as 'hysteria of the stomach' or 'inflammation of the uterus'.

So-called treatments included choking women's necks, drinking urine and inserting a tampon of powdered fox testicles.

After the Witchcraft Act of 1604 in England, it was common for women with gynaecological disorders to be tortured and killed. It was a difficult time to be a woman full stop, let alone a woman with an invisible illness that might cause her to moan and writhe around in pain. During one documented trial, Dutch physician Johannes Weyer, called as an expert witness, tried to persuade the court that rather than being in cahoots with the devil, the woman in question was suffering from a 'bodily disease like all other medical conditions'.

'Don't you know that these poor women have suffered enough?' he said at the trial. 'Can you think of a misery anywhere in the world that is worse than theirs? If they do seem to merit punishment, I assure you, their illness alone is enough.'

I am moved by this testimony, a male doctor who had authority, daring to speak up against injustice at a time when so few did. Of course, he was then accused of witchcraft himself.

By the eighteenth century, French clinicians were performing autopsies on women who had died from sudden intense pain during menstruation, in what is now believed to be cases of ruptured ovarian cysts. Austrian pathologist Carl von Rokitansky was the first to microscopically discover endometriosis in 1860, but treatments were not for the faint-hearted. They included 'ovary compressors', sulphuric acid, turpentine or mercury applied directly into the womb and leeches shoved into the cervix. Sometimes leeches were accidentally left behind.

With the advent of surgery came a terrifying period of mortality for endometriosis patients. At first there was the 'twist and tear' method, followed by the 'clawing out' technique in which surgeons would use blunt scissors or their own fingernails to remove the lesions. Unsurprisingly, the death rate from blood loss or infection soared, to between 70 and 90 per cent. Today endometriosis is not considered to be a fatal disease, but women do still die from associated complications.

Every now and then a 'cure' or 'new treatment' for endometriosis appears in the news and friends will forward me the link. But if you read the fine print it's usually another medication that shuts down production of oestrogen from the ovaries, preventing ovulation, and therefore is no good to anyone who is hoping to conceive. Many of these new drugs also have side effects, are not designed to be taken long-term, and symptoms usually recur when the medication is stopped. While there are some promising studies going on, it takes years for trials to evolve from experimental to prescribable. Therefore, as it stands, many of us are staring down the barrel of living with a progressive disease for the foreseeable future, which is incredibly depressing.

In January 2021, after years of daily pain, Trinity Lillian Graves, an eighteen-year-old from Chicago, was diagnosed with endometriosis. Three months later she texted her mum:

> I'm in so much pain I want to die.

Within six months she had taken her own life.

The BBC surveyed 13,500 women with endometriosis and found that around half had experienced suicidal thoughts. Trinity's mother, Sarah, wrote a moving blog post to raise awareness about her daughter's story.

> When Trinity experienced a dip in pain, she'd emerge! Bubbly, funny, teasing (her sisters), cooking, creating, inventing, sewing, crocheting, working on photography, making candles, soap, and jewelry, and cleaning, organizing, and engaging with friends.

We are not just people in pain, we are creatives and makers and lovers and our lives are full of potential. But our outsides do not always match up with our insides. If we contain multitudes then some are glutted with paradox. I am not just this person, ravaged by the faulty tissue I've been stuffed with. I also work, I walk, I dream. I go to brunches and parties and weddings. I get on trains and planes and dance the night away at music festivals. I pet dogs in the park and I play tennis. And sometimes I need painkillers and hot water bottles to get through the day. Sometimes I pace around the house with a restless fervour, like a dog circling its bed, unable to get comfortable. Some days I spend hours researching new treatments and other days I write about my pain to try and give it some purpose.

In the blog post, Sarah, Trinity's mum, continued:

This is serious. Endometriosis destroys lives. Ladies, if you can, please have the courage to tell the graphic version of your story. Tell it, write it, share it, photograph it, and post it.

So that is what I am doing. For Jahmby, for Aubrion, for Trinity, and for all the women who were subjected to abuse and torture hundreds of years ago. For the next generation of girls and women who deserve a full life, not a half-sick one.

Endometriosis is a mystery, they say, an enigma. I have read it over and over again. Its causes may be unknown, but that does not mean they are unknowable. It wasn't very long ago that we didn't know about germs or blood types. We used to know very little about cholera and syphilis and now they are easily treatable. We have made massive strides in cancer treatment over the last forty years. We put our heads together and created a Covid vaccine in ten months. So why is endometriosis treatment stuck in the dark ages?

We need to talk to women. We need to do trials with women. We need to stop excluding women from trials because their hormone cycles make it more time-consuming or inconvenient to analyse results. The pros are greater than the cons. If we don't fund this properly we are letting down another generation of two hundred million girls and women. And that's not good enough.

Blood

Definition

1. A red liquid pumped by the heart
2. Family background; descent or lineage
3. Life, or the taking of life

By late 2020, I was in a new relationship with a charming and boyishly handsome man called James. We'd worked on the crime series together – the one I had been filming when the donor joined the DNA website – and I'd confided in him throughout my unravelling identity crisis. He was a great listener, made me laugh and we shared similar views on the world. James enjoyed poetry, arthouse films and was a stronger advocate of feminism than most women I know. We went to art exhibitions, read Orwell to each other and wrote long emails during lockdown. I was intoxicated by how quickly our connection had developed, and how deep it went. If love were a video game, it felt like I'd tapped into a new level I hadn't known existed. When the world shut down during the pandemic, it felt like ours was opening up. I wanted to hear his views on things and he wanted to hear mine. Everything – nature, language, intimacy – felt infinitely more alive and possible.

James knew I felt pressured by my diagnosis to have children in the next few years, so when we started dating I was relieved that he seemed sympathetic and understanding. In the early months of our relationship we talked about our visions of the future, with his involving some 'little nippers running around' and taking them travelling. When he told me I would make a good mother my belly fluttered. He wanted to move more slowly than I did, but I was excited about our future.

It wasn't long before I came off the pill, a decision that James supported. I'd been on it for twelve years and wanted to give my body a break, allowing my hormones to settle down before trying for a baby in the future. On my fertile days – tracked by an app that measured my temperature every morning – we used the pull-out method, and on the other days we just took our chances.

'What if I accidentally got pregnant?' I asked him.

'We'd make it work,' he replied. 'It would be an adventure.'

My heart swelled. His spontaneous attitude to life was one of the things I loved about him. While Sam had seemed to assume that starting a family while in a relatively new relationship in his early thirties might ruin his life and career, James appeared to picture an 'accident' much more positively.

A few months before James and I started dating, I found myself lying on the bathroom floor of my parents' house. I knew I needed help but couldn't bring myself to ask for it. The day was getting late and I watched the low April sun begin her handover to the night shift. The sky was the colour of a conch shell; pastel pink whipped into smooth curves of creamy clouds. Just weeks earlier, the Covid pandemic had shut down the world, and my life trajectory had taken a nosedive. Almost overnight I lost my job, broke up with Sam and moved back in with my parents. It wasn't quite what I had envisioned for my twenty-eight-year-old self.

And now I was on the verge of fainting. My own body was thwarting my plans. I had fainted enough times in my life to know the warning signs, but even though my family were only downstairs, I couldn't tell them what I was doing. Still, I knew that fainting and hitting my head in a locked bathroom would be worse. I didn't know what to do. I laid my head on the carpeted step and prayed I would bleed some more.

For over an hour I had been attempting to squeeze a small vial's worth of blood from my hand. I had tried all the tricks: a hot shower, star jumps, tying something around my arm, but the blood was congealing at my fingertips too fast. Three different digits had now been nicked with the single-use prick tests and I had only one left. Just a couple more drops would fill the tube up to the line, but I knew I would faint if I kept going; the silverfish speckles in my peripheral vision told me that I was dangerously close. Outside, the cake batter clouds were turning grey, the moon now in full view; a gaunt, waxing crescent. I couldn't shut myself in the bathroom all evening.

For over a year the family secret had been mentally tugging at me and to quiet it down I had decided to donate my own eggs to a stranger. Having done so much research about the process for the TV show I was pitching, I knew there was a shortage of egg donors in the UK. I weighed up the pros and cons and decided it would be worth it to help someone else, as well as a fitting form of closure for me.

In an ideal world I would have waited until I'd had my own children before donating, as many donors do, but I didn't want to risk being too old by then, since egg donors must be under the age of thirty-five. Ultimately I figured if I was just washing my eggs down the toilet every month and not using them right now, someone else might as well be. Sending off a blood sample in the post was the first step, but I didn't want to tell my family what I was doing until the agency had confirmed that I was a suitable donor. An online search told me that more than 50 per cent of egg donors who applied were rejected. As well as being under thirty-five, most clinics require donors to be non-smokers, have a good ovarian reserve, a healthy body mass index and be able to provide a thorough medical history.

A few weeks earlier I had found an egg donation agency online and sent them an email. A nice lady called me back the next day and we had a long chat over the phone. I told her about my own history and reasons for wanting to donate. She said that of all the donors she had spoken to over the years, it sounded like I had the most in-depth understanding and empathy for the recipients because of my own story. The next step, she said, was to send me an at-home blood test kit to check my AMH level (Anti-Mullerian hormone) as it is a good indicator of how many eggs you have left. She said if the number was too low it might compromise my future fertility so it would not be in my interest to donate.

It was eighteen months after my endometriosis diagnosis and, approaching thirty, I wanted to know how fast my clock was ticking. I saw donating as a chance to get a fertility MOT. Since all my TV work had fallen through due to the pandemic and I was relying on a couple of small ghostwriting jobs for the foreseeable, it was a bonus that I would get paid £750 in expenses to donate.

Back in the bathroom, I was trying to stay conscious. It wasn't the first time I'd fainted in there. One morning, when I was fifteen, I awoke to the sound of my sister, Ruth, screaming. I darted to the bathroom to find her sat on the toilet seat swaddled in her bathrobe, sobbing. Mum often left her clothes in a folded pile on the floor and Ruth had accidentally stepped on her belt buckle while getting out of the shower. The metal prong had stabbed deep into the fleshy arch of her sole. When she yelled, Mum ran in and yanked it out. As I arrived, Ruth lifted her foot to show me, revealing a bluish bruise around a small puncture wound. Surprisingly, there was no blood.

I asked her what had happened and as she started talking I caught sight of my drab reflection in the mirror. I don't know if it was the headrush of running out of bed, the gore of the story or some kind of sisterly empathy, but I lost consciousness.

I woke up to bodies staring down at me and cold tiles cooling my cheeks. My head pounded to make sense of the new perspective. Why was everyone so far away? I had stumbled backwards into the shower, down an eight-inch step and my legs were above me. The house phone started ringing; Dad was calling from work. Everything was chaos. A sharp headache drummed my skull.

'Call 911, call 911!' shouted Joe, who'd watched too many American cartoons. That's not the right number, we told him later.

Eventually I climbed to my feet, holding the base of my skull, feeling for cracks. Ruth limped out of the bathroom. Looking like casualties at the scene of a car crash, we headed back to our rooms, put on our uniforms and caught the bus to school as normal. The Coxon way is to carry on.

Finding myself enclosed within the same four walls, I mustered the strength to sit up and try my finger one last time, squeezing ferociously along the tired bones and scraping the red treacle over the lip of the world's smallest test tube. But it was not enough. Moonlight blinked into the room; it was time to give up. I packed away the box, buried it in a drawer in my bedroom and resolved to try again in the morning.

The next day I managed to fill the tube to the line, just, and post it without my family noticing. A couple of weeks later the woman from the egg donor agency called again. She told me my AMH level was on the low side but enough to donate. I didn't know whether to be concerned or relieved. Next I would have to fill out an online profile – to give them a sense of 'my personality and character' – and upload two photographs, a recent one and another from when I was a small child. Only the agency would see the current photo, to help them match me appearance-wise, while the picture of me as a child would be seen by my recipient family.

Within a few weeks, I was matched. The recipient was informed about my endometriosis diagnosis and decided to continue with the match. Because of the laws around anonymity, they couldn't tell me anything other than that the recipient was a single woman in her forties.

'You have a lot in common,' the woman said. 'If you knew each other I have no doubt you'd be friends.'

A few months later, I attended a compulsory online counselling session. The counsellor was warm and empathetic as we discussed the psychological impact of the process. I mentioned that among my reasons for donating was my discovery that I was donor-conceived myself and wanted to pay it forward. As she delved further, I admitted that I had not told anyone in my family that I was planning to donate my eggs.

'When donating eggs,' she explained, 'it's very important that the donor doesn't change their mind at the last minute. There have been instances when a loved one has found out and reacted so badly that the donor has pulled out of the procedure.'

'Oh,' I said.

'Of course, it's hugely disruptive for the recipient, and a situation that everyone wants to avoid.'

I nodded. 'I'm definitely not going to change my mind.'

'What about your parents? Occasionally we find that a parent of a donor feels like their daughter is "giving away" their grandchild, and tries to stop the donation.'

'I understand,' I said. 'But I think it would be pretty hypocritical of my parents to prevent me, their donor-conceived child, from donating.' I looked out the window. 'I'm reluctant to bring it up with them because it might stir up some difficult feelings around the family secret and stuff.'

'You don't have to tell them; ultimately it is up to you. But I would strongly suggest you think about it. Maybe just your mum?'

'Okay,' I sighed, knowing she was right. 'I think I'll tell my mum.'

Belly

Definition

1. Stomach
2. Womb
3. The underside of a place

Three years into our relationship, James and I went on holiday to Thailand. I had been looking forward to the adventure, but a disturbing combination of an endometriosis flare-up and long-haul flight constipation had left my body particularly swollen and sore. My belly felt like a hand-pumped balloon, so taut that a cough might puncture it. My intestines twisted into the shape of a sausage dog.

We were staying on a beautiful island, embedded between mangroves, and every morning James suggested we walk to the beach to swim, paddleboard or snorkel. Of course, how lovely! That's what holidays are for! But all I wanted to do was lie on the bed in our hotel room, read and mope. I couldn't face wearing a bikini or swimsuit when I felt like this. The crop-tops and figure-hugging dresses I'd packed a few days earlier seemed tyrannical to me now. If I wore them outside the room people might think I was pregnant. How wrong they would be. How awkward to tell them, no, this bloating is likely a symptom of my infertility, actually.

When I get sad about these things, living inside a body that feels achingly out of my control, I think of women I admire and lean into their stories for comfort and strength. Maya Angelou, Oprah Winfrey, Elizabeth Gilbert, Glennon Doyle, Gretchen Rubin. I have never seen photos of any of these women wearing bikinis. The reason I respect them is because they are brilliant – writers, thinkers, activists, artists – not because of the size of their bellies or the state of their reproductive systems.

At the age of twenty-four, I met Ruth for a five-week trip around Central America – after she'd sailed from Southampton to the Caribbean in a tall ship, monitoring whales – and we put Mexico City on our list of stops. With Mexico's reputation in the media for drugs and gang violence, I did not have high expectations, but the city was sprawling and vibrant, like an exploded orange dahlia. Creativity and potential seemed to be at the heart of everything: food, art, film, life. I noticed that everywhere we went we saw the same face: on postcards and graffiti, in airports and down alleyways. We had arrived from Cuba, a place still humming its own nostalgic love ballad to Che Guevara, a face so integral to Cubans' very existence, but this monobrowed woman – so poised and impervious – waltzed into my consciousness more slowly. I'm embarrassed to say that I didn't know who Frida Kahlo was. It wasn't until two years later, in 2018, when I visited an exhibition of Kahlo's personal belongings at the V&A in London – the first of its kind outside Mexico – that I became truly enamoured by her story.

Throughout most of her life, Kahlo wore long, sweeping skirts and wide Tehuana dresses with traditional Mexican huipiles (beautiful, embroidered boxy tunics) draped with fringed shawls and bold-coloured jewellery. Her playful nature and pride in her indigenous Mexican heritage clearly influenced her appearance, but this style of clothing also allowed her to cover up the scars from her many spinal surgeries and hide her atrophied (and later, prosthetic) leg, caused by childhood polio. Kahlo, we seem to forget, was a disabled artist. Today she is known mostly for her self-portraits and photographs of her face – often adorned with flowers or animals – and that enigmatic facial expression. However, her art had a much darker side too. In some of her portraits Kahlo paints herself nude, but rather than evoking sensuality or eroticism, it is her pain and suffering that is exposed: a medical abortion, miscarriage or bleeding to death, after being stabbed by her lover. 'In Frida's work,' her biographer Raquel Tibol writes, 'oil paint mixes with the blood of her inner monologue.' Her paintings were provocative, radical images at the time, and are no less so today.

My favourite of all Kahlo's artworks is an oil painting called *The Broken Column*, in which her naked torso is split in two, revealing the tubal cavity where her spine should be, as if she has been hollowed by an apple corer. Her upper body and breasts are encased in a surgical corset made of steel and covered in white fabric. Tears freckle her cheeks and her flesh is littered with nails, piercing her all over like a human dartboard. A martyred saint perhaps; crucified and maimed by stigmata, everywhere but her hands. The Ionic column that replaces her spine, and props her up, is eroding and dangerously splintered. The white sheet that covers her from the hips down is brushed with blood stains. Kahlo's expression is sullen and resigned, both intense and mute. She stares straight at us, but her eyes are glazed. This pain is not new. She knows we cannot help her.

The way we feel on the inside so often reflects how we see the outside world. The previous year James and I spent a few weeks in Greece. I was feeling burned out from work and blistered by my inflamed insides, desperate to start trying for a baby before it was too late. It was a very hot day in Athens when we planned to walk the steep steps of the Acropolis. As we headed towards the entrance, I told James I needed to stop for a second. My belly was swollen and griping.

'I hate this,' I said, leaning over an ancient wall. 'It hurts so much and every time it just feels like a big fat reminder.'

'A reminder of what?' he asked.

'That it might be difficult to have kids. And that we haven't even started trying yet.'

In my fantasy-brain, this was the moment when he would hug me, tell me he'd given it some thought and decided that we should finally start trying. But he looked off into the distance, then back at me.

'I'm not ready,' he said.

I sat down, aware of the tourists walking past, licking their ice creams and holding their children's hands.

'What makes you feel not ready?' I asked.

'I don't know. I don't really have an answer.'

'Okay.' I took a deep breath. 'When do you think you might be ready?'

'I can't really say. But not for another year, at least.'

I heaved in shock and turned away from him. The thought of another year before we even started trying winded me. I didn't understand how he could want children with me but not take into account the body that would be carrying them, and the mind too. My mental health was suffering from years of endometriosis hollowing me out, while watching friend after friend fall pregnant. I knew that finding out the full extent of my parents' fertility issues had set off a fire alarm inside my own head, but I also knew we could be in the same boat as them. Nothing was guaranteed. My body might cause problems, or it might not. Yet there was no urgency for James. Like most people approaching thirty, he was assuming his fertility was fine and functional, with no evidence either way. And I understood. I wished I could be as blasé about the future as him. I wished I wasn't running on a treadmill that was going twice the speed of everyone else's.

No one should be pushed into a decision like having children and commit to something so permanent when they don't feel ready. I respected James's stance, but I felt deflated; all the joy of being on holiday wheezing out of me. As we hiked up the steps of the Acropolis, my head and belly throbbed. I needed to lie down. There was nowhere in the shade so I lay on a hot stone bench in the vicious sun. Within seconds a security guard shouted and demanded I get up. It felt cruel. We got up and traipsed the rest of the hot steep hill in silence.

We took the obligatory photos in front of the old ruins; I smiled and sucked my belly in. I posed for a playful picture, squatting down with my palms facing upwards like I was trying to lift up some giant columns; carrying the weight of the world.

A few days later, we went kayaking and despite floating on the most dazzling, glassy-blue sea, I couldn't stop crying. I felt so low and alone. And then I felt guilty for feeling sad when I should be happy and grateful, not ruining another day of our holiday. James later joked that I had created a new sport: 'cry-aking'. He did his best to comfort me and take my mind off things, but it's hard to feel comforted by the person who is hurting your heart. I didn't have the language to communicate how I was feeling to my friends or family. I wasn't infertile or miscarrying – the kind of grief we understand better – I was in limbo, stuck, waiting, longing; unable to start trying.

The landscape behind Kahlo in *The Broken Column* is beige, barren and ruptured, like cardboard ripped up in a sudden rage. Above it a simple blue sky. Kahlo is fragmented but somehow held together, still alive. The sky and sea carry on, oblivious to her inner struggles. Like so many of her self-portraits, *The Broken Column* reflects the enduring agony Kahlo experienced in her personal life, both physically and psychologically. The polio she contracted as a child and the injuries she suffered from a bus accident at the age of eighteen are well-documented, but the subsequent effects of these injuries on her fertility, and her deep desire for children, are lesser known despite being a prominent theme in her work. Look more closely and you will see that her paintings are brimming with breastfeeding, umbilical cords, dried blood and unborn babies.

Kahlo was pregnant at least three times in her life, but none of her children were carried to term. Her body would not allow it. Doctors now believe her infertility to have been caused by Asherman's syndrome, the presence of scar tissue in the womb that often gives rise to recurrent miscarriage. The extra tissue takes up too much space and can cause the walls of the womb to fuse together, stifling the growth of any foetus. For Kahlo it's likely the scar tissue developed as a result of the bus accident she experienced as a teenager, when a metal handrail impaled her abdomen. Her fertility problems were likely compounded by her subsequent miscarriages and medically necessary terminations, the aftermath of which involved scraping inside her womb to remove dead tissue, but in turn created more scar tissue.

In letters to her doctor, Kahlo writes how she had so looked forward to having 'a little Dieguito' (a baby with her husband Diego) and had cried a lot about the thought of not having children. She goes on to say that she had always been jealous of Diego's first wife for her ability to bear his two daughters. Kahlo's infertility haunted her but so did something else: Diego did not want children with her. He'd abandoned the ones he had from his previous marriage and made it clear he did not want any more. 'I suffered two grave accidents in my life,' she wrote. 'One in which a streetcar knocked me down ... The other accident is Diego. Diego was by far the worst.'

Along with his recurring infidelities, including, most devastatingly, with Kahlo's own sister, she must have felt deeply isolated in her struggle to conceive. 'I paint myself because I am alone,' she wrote. It's hard falling in love with someone who doesn't want the same things that you do.

Kahlo underwent over thirty surgeries during her life. Between them she was required to wear orthopaedic corsets because her spine was too weak to support itself. The corsets helped her to sit and stand, but she also felt they were a 'punishment', a reminder that she would forever be imprisoned within and restricted by her own body. The fabric corsets were white so, naturally, Kahlo painted over them, her body literally a canvas. On one of them, she painted a red hammer and sickle, parallel to her heart. Below it, a foetus curled up in the womb.

The child she would never hold.

Ghost

Definition

1. The spirit of a dead person
2. To end a relationship suddenly by stopping all communication
3. Someone who ghostwrites

On Frida Kahlo's forty-fifth birthday, a little girl called Hilary was born across the ocean in England. She would go on to become an enormously successful writer and double Booker prizewinner, but, like Kahlo, infertility haunted her. For Hilary Mantel, it was severe endometriosis that took away her choice to have children. By her late twenties, endometriosis had become an 'evil web' in her life, a 'scraping and chiselling' that hurt 'every part of [her] body'. Having been misdiagnosed for years as suffering from a mental illness, she was finally admitted to hospital for surgery to determine the cause of her chronic pain. When she woke up from the anaesthetic she discovered that they had removed 'her reproductive apparatus', namely her womb, ovaries and part of her bowels. A surgical menopause. She was twenty-seven.

'Abruptly I lost my fertility and, in some ways, lost myself,' she wrote. 'It was a case of waking up with no choice.'

In her memoir *Giving Up the Ghost*, Mantel writes movingly about the children she never had. 'Their lives start long before birth, long before conception, and if they are aborted or miscarried or simply fail to materialise at all, they become ghosts within our lives.'

In the early years of their marriage, Mantel and her husband had mused on a name for a future daughter: Catriona. 'I assumed I would be able to have Catriona at a time of my choosing,' she wrote. 'I didn't know she would always be a ghost of possibility, a paper baby, a person who slipped between the lines.'

Mantel was diagnosed with endometriosis in the late 1970s and wasn't offered IVF or egg freezing before her surgery; it was not yet available. Doctors simply removed the body parts affected by the disease and that was that. Unfortunately, removing Mantel's affected organs did not rid her of endometriosis and she continued to struggle with its symptoms and the terrible side effects of inappropriately prescribed medication for years afterwards.

Mantel was born eleven months after my mother. It strikes me now that had my mother spoken up about her symptoms earlier, before trying to conceive, she too might have been operated on. She too might have been left wombless and childless. My siblings and I might have been ghost children.

In her fifties, Mantel wrote a moving article for *The Times*: 'I was taken aback by my feelings recently when a friend became a grandmother. I'm haunted by the ghosts of the children that never were and by the ghost of the mother I never was.'

In September 2022 Mantel passed away suddenly after suffering a stroke. Tributes poured in from every corner of the earth. One tweet read:

'A true Goddess. Her book Giving Up the Ghost is the most searing portrait of living in a female body that can be read. Her work is eternal.'

It was written by actor, director and writer Lena Dunham, most well-known for her hit television series *Girls*. Dunham was diagnosed with endometriosis in her twenties and, after nine surgeries, wrote publicly about opting for a hysterectomy as a last resort, at the age of thirty-one. In an article for *Vogue* she said, 'With pain like this, I will never be able to be anyone's mother.'

I know the feeling. There are days when the condition, like a parasite, sucks so much from you; energy, patience, hope. And yet, to remove the cause of the pain is to remove the ability to create a future we desire. It is this 'illusion of choice', as Dunham has described it, that paralyses many of us. The options for making living more bearable are often in direct conflict with the opportunity to have a family.

Dunham elected to have her uterus, cervix and one affected ovary removed. There are days I want to remove my temperamental organs too. Days when I want to scream: 'Fine, I'm leaving you!' like a maddened lover. On these days, resentment recruits revenge and I imagine my organs – antagonistic and aflame – finally detached from me, lying on a cold steel operating table, then tossed into the clinical waste bin.

But I want children, I know it in my bones. There are plenty of people who don't, and I will defend their right to decide that for themselves till the end of eternity. But I do. There are other ways to have children of course – surrogacy and adoption, for example – but I've always felt envious of pregnant bodies. I'd love to carry a child and feel that bond, experience the chaos and calm of pregnancy and birth, breastfeed if I can. Like Dunham, I want to know what 'nine months of complete togetherness could feel like'.

Dunham 'never had a single doubt about having children' and after her hysterectomy she wrote about desiring it more than ever. 'The moment I lost my fertility I started searching for a baby.'

When something is taken away from you, it can make you want it more. As my decision about 'when' to have children became an 'if', I couldn't stop thinking about it. What if I can't? What if I leave it too late? For me, the looming prospect of infertility has become a kind of obsession, a scramble for control.

After the hysterectomy, Dunham discovered there were still ways she could become a biological mother. Her options were limited but not impossible. Her recent break-up with her boyfriend made things trickier, but she took her window of opportunity and underwent fertility treatment to collect eggs from her remaining ovary. The eggs were then fertilised using sperm donated by a friend.

'I was another cocky woman-to-be,' she wrote, 'sure that I would have what I wanted because I wanted it. Because I had always gotten it. What started as wanting to carry the child of the man I loved became wanting to have a child with a man who was willing to help me have one. Soon that became hiring a lawyer to draft a contract for a sperm-donor friend and calling a surrogate who came highly recommended by another celebrity.'

But our lives don't always pan out as we hope. Ten years ago, when my flatmates and I were musing about who would get married and have children first, of course there had to be someone who came last, and it turned out to be me. Many more of my friends are parents now too and while I relish their joys and celebrate at their hen parties, weddings and baby showers, I'm also gripped by an underlying sadness that my own life has not taken any of those shapes yet.

Until my late twenties I had not given much thought to endometriosis, sperm donors, or hysterectomies. I didn't even really know what they were. Then they all dropped on top of me at once. As I read about the experiences of celebrities like Dunham, I don't know if I'm comforted or alarmed to realise that even the most successful people in the world can brush up against barriers of ill health and the limitations of the human body. Money, connections and admiration can't get you everything.

Unfortunately none of Dunham's six eggs developed into a viable embryo. 'There is a lot you can correct in life,' she wrote, 'you can end a relationship, get sober, get serious, say sorry – but you can't force the universe to give you a baby that your body has told you all along was an impossibility.' Despite its major advances, modern fertility treatment does not guarantee success. 'I was meant for the job,' she wrote, 'but I didn't pass the interview.'

I often think about the people who wanted to be parents and tried for years, perhaps decades, only to be forced to accept that nature would not allow it. I think of the hundreds of generations of ghost children who never lived beyond a dream, a longing, a twinkle in their parents' eye. All the children who were deeply wanted but will never be.

We talk about the 'pram in the hall' affecting women's lives and careers, but what about the ghost pram in the hall? The alternate lives of parenthood that haunt us?

Despite her own experiences with infertility, Hilary Mantel felt that reproductive technologies were a 'mixed' blessing. For anonymous sperm donation in particular, she was not a glowing supporter.

'Women with infertile partners conceive with the help of sperm donors, usually anonymous: that is to say, they have a child with a man they have never set eyes on,' she wrote. 'I suppose I should say I respect their choice. But I don't, not really. I think it's weird.'

So, unfortunately, according to Mantel – an author I deeply respect – I am *weird*. Or at least, the product of weird decision-making. Never meet your heroes, they say, but perhaps also do not ask them about your right to exist. But alas, I am not offended. Mantel was writing in 2003, a time when stigma reigned more mightily, and in any case sperm donation was not something she necessarily needed or was offered. Had it been, who knows whether she may have felt differently. Either way, I should address my own prejudices here. Mantel's view on sperm donation was pretty much the way I felt a few years ago, before I learned about my own origins. I thought it was a bit weird, too. I think a part of me still does.

Many of us imagine serendipity and romance to be at the heart of our procreation stories, but as a storyteller, I'm aware that often the most satisfying endings arise after some conflict and struggle. A baby brought into this world through medical procedures and the genetic code of strangers, in a pond of personal grief, may not make for a beautiful story, but I am choosing to write it that way. There is still poetry in it. Assisted reproductive technology, the clue is in the name. We are art. I am choosing to reframe these stories to help myself and others see that our genetic make-up is just one part of our story, as unique and mysterious and miraculous as anyone else's. And I think Hilary Mantel would approve of that.

We are lucky to be a generation with many more options than our mothers and grandmothers. These unorthodox journeys to parenthood are not what anyone imagines for themselves; they are not chosen or sought after. They are often difficult, emotionally wrought paths that test people's physical and mental limits. But they offer hope, only afforded to us in the last few decades, after thousands of years of heartache. Scientists have vastly improved the prognosis of procreation, allowing those stymied by an array of biological obstacles to have the families they yearn for. It has meant that millions of 'ghost' children exist today. I am one of them. My children might be too.

When I was at high school we learned about the case of a woman called Diane Blood in an ethics lesson. In the mid-1990s, Blood was called 'sick' and 'strange' for wanting a family with the man she'd been with for twelve years. Diane and her husband Stephen had been trying, but it would take three years and two landmark court battles before she was allowed to conceive their child by IVF. Why? Because Stephen was dead.

There have always been children born with ghost parents: fathers who died in the months between conception and birth, and mothers who died in childbirth. But since the 1980s there have been an increasing number of children conceived from the sperm of men who were already dead. Some, knowing they were ill, froze their sperm and granted permission for it to be used after their death. Others did not, leaving an ethical minefield, literally, in their wake.

But what kind of people attempt to carry on a person's lineage after they're gone and why? For Diane Blood, the future she had planned with her husband included children and she didn't see why she couldn't continue with that plan.

'Yes, I'd lost my husband, I'd lost a huge part of my life that was irreplaceable,' she said, 'but I didn't need to lose it all.' The British courts argued that because Blood did not have written consent from her husband, she was not entitled to his sperm. At the age of thirty, Stephen contracted bacterial meningitis, fell into a coma and died within a week, something his wife was obviously not expecting nor could prepare for. But while the court argued that it was illegal to store Stephen's sperm, they did not rule that it was illegal to take it, and a bizarre legal fight ensued with the Human Fertilisation and Embryology Authority.

'What I found hard to grasp,' Blood said, 'was that I could have the sperm of an anonymous donor, even one who was dead, but not my own husband.'

Eventually the high court agreed she could take his sperm to a fertility clinic abroad. A Belgian clinic offered to help and over the following years Blood gave birth to two sons.

Since the start of the Gaza war in October 2023, an increasing number of bereaved parents have been requesting sperm from the bodies of their sons or partners to be extracted and frozen. When a soldier dies in combat and the dreaded news is delivered to the family, these days they may also be presented with a question: would they like his sperm retrieved? The process must be done within seventy-two hours of death, ideally within twenty-four. It involves making a small incision in the testicle and removing a piece of tissue from which sperm cells can be collected and used in fertility treatment like any other sperm; creating the children of ghosts.

Alongside making documentaries, I have also been a professional ghostwriter for the past ten years. In a way it's like being a surrogate mother. The story (the embryo) comes from the client – I write down the words, grow the foetus and give birth to it – but the book (the baby) belongs to them. The books I have written are mostly memoirs that involve shaping negative experiences into something more positive. Cancer diagnoses, suicide bereavement, rape, parental abandonment. There is no shortage of sadness in the world and most of us would agree that revisiting these experiences and contouring them – through writing, art or campaigning – can give people a much-needed sense of purpose. How we remember and record these things can positively impact how we move on with our lives after trauma or tragedy. It gives me great pleasure to watch as the clients I work with start to feel lighter and more confident in themselves once their story takes shape. I find they are also more compelled to advocate for others as a result too.

But the reality is that sharing our stories can both alleviate and exacerbate shame. Often it's a dance, from day to day, between the two. When we open ourselves up to others we have no control over how they will react. Indeed, the public response can shift depending on the trends, headlines and political opinions of the time. It really is no wonder that my parents kept their conception journey a secret from everyone they knew. In the eighties and nineties, IVF alone was a big, bouncy newcomer that divided public opinion. Newspapers at the time showed mocked-up babies preserved in glass jars like freak-show curiosities. Louise Brown's birth brought ripples of hope but also tidal waves of controversy around the world. News spread about the rise in 'test-tube babies' as if we were mutations, or clones, or entirely undeserving of a womb to call home. My own grandmother believed IVF created 'monster babies'. It was many years before people began to accept that babies conceived by IVF were just normal children.

Had my parents been more open about their journey to parenthood, who knows what other people might have said to try and deter them. *Give up the ghost. Don't interfere with nature. Children are a gift from God. Don't force it. It's not meant to be.* I wish I could say that these kinds of comments have been relegated to the dark ages of the past, but I see them in social media comments every week.

> Sad, selfish people.
>
> It is nature's way of telling you something is not right.
>
> People should take it as a sign that if they can't conceive naturally then maybe children aren't for them.
>
> Infertility is not an illness so should be paid for privately.
>
> Get a dog instead.

It is easy to condemn the choices of others when we have not experienced those same struggles ourselves. These comments are likely from people who have conceived their own children easily, do not want children or are yet to have their own fertility tested. Ignorance may be bliss, but it can make people brutal.

Since the Roe vs Wade abortion rights were overturned in the United States in June 2022, campaigners and journalists have warned that some Republicans are now 'waging war on IVF' and 'coming for birth control and fertility treatments'.

'Children,' says the United States Conference of Catholic Bishops, 'should be begotten not made.' Despite being pro-life, the Catholic Church – of which there are 1.3 billion members in the world – has taken a strong and unequivocal stance against assisted reproduction, and IVF in particular, declaring it 'immoral' and against the 'human dignity of our offspring'.

In 2010, Catholic bishops in Poland branded IVF 'the younger sister of eugenics', while a diocese in the US recently described it as an 'intrinsic evil, flowing from the decision to allow our offspring to be "manufactured"'. Are we no more than products of a corrupted industry? The result of a science experiment? We may be 'man-made', but I believe we are products of nature too. Evolution favours experimentation.

The Church's reasonings are related to the 'sinful' masturbation involved in collecting sperm samples, the notion that sexual intercourse should not be for any other purpose than procreation and the belief that life begins at conception, so the discarding of any unused or non-viable embryos is murder.

It is worth saying that, in comparison, other denominations of the Christian church, along with the religions of Islam, Hinduism, Judaism, Buddhism and Mormonism, hold more flexible views on assisted reproduction and IVF, provided that the couple are married and it is their own egg and sperm used. I am pleased about this, but it still means that most religions on this earth believe that my siblings and I should not have been born.

I find it peculiar that society – be it the government, media, religious groups or the average Joe – feels the need to wade in so heavily on an individual's medical decisions when they relate to fertility. Most people do not hold an opinion on the latest techniques for heart surgery or hip replacements; they lack the specialist knowledge and most have not undertaken difficult decisions associated with those particular procedures. It is left up to the doctors and the patients to decide what is best, medically and ethically, in each individual's circumstances. But the same cannot be said for fertility treatment, about which it appears everyone is entitled to an opinion. We tend not to question whether heart surgery is 'selfish' or 'immoral', words that have long been associated with fertility treatment. Is it selfish to want a heart that works? A womb that works? To request that our tubes be unblocked, and if not, bypassed by some other technique? Are arteries and sperm ducts or fallopian tubes really so different?

If we preserve somebody's eggs or sperm before chemotherapy, does that count as fertility treatment? If we save somebody's life through surgery or medication when they are young and they go on to have children in the future, is that kind of medical intervention acceptable? Matters of fertility are not black and white. Our bodies and lifestyles change over time, diseases progress or disappear. We may be able to conceive naturally when we are eighteen but not by the time we are thirty. Does this mean we should have children while we are young instead of waiting until we are financially secure and emotionally mature?

Diane Blood's landmark case was controversial. Some members of the public supported her, while others compared her to Dolly the cloned sheep, called her a fanatic and said she was unable to move on from her husband's death.

'One does not have to agree with her decision to have her husband's children, nor even to like her,' wrote Emma Brockes in the *Guardian* in 2004. 'One has only to agree that the decision was hers to make and not the HFEA's.'

Interestingly, Blood describes herself as a Christian. 'The matter of conception,' she said, 'I felt that was in God's hands. Whereas before that, it was man getting in the way saying, "No, you can't even try." Nobody can say whether they can have a baby or not, but I think they have the right to try.'

Thirty years ago my parents, and others like them, went against the grain, making decisions that were, and evidently still are, controversial. But they did so with the support and guidance of some fantastically skilled, pioneering and discreet medical professionals. I am grateful to them all. Together they formed a picket line for progress, a rebellion against the arbitrary constraints of 'nature'. In the words of T.S. Eliot, they dared to disturb the universe.

The Catholic Church argues that by conceiving through IVF 'new life is not engendered through an act of love between husband and wife'. But I believe there can be just as much, if not more love in the process of fertility treatment. Anyone can have sex, but IVF is arduous and painstaking. There are no tests or tick-lists for couples to complete before getting frisky after a bottle of wine, yet going through fertility treatment requires months of honest conversations, medical consultations and signatures on dotted lines; ongoing pledges of each partner's time, patience and trust. It is sending off vials of bodily fluids to be assessed and analysed; liquid commitment, sharp scratches of hope.

I choose to believe there was boundless love and kindness in the room when my siblings and I were nurtured from individual cells in our Petri dishes. A whole team willing us to grow. They say it takes a village to raise a child, but sometimes it takes a team of medical professionals to conceive one.

I am one of the 'test-tube babies'; one of the guinea pigs that scientists were lauded and lambasted for, gambling with the game of life. One of the inconceivables who now make up more than 1 per cent of the population. In any other century we could not have existed. Through sharing stories like mine, I hope the stigma and shame can be moulded into something more meaningful. I hope to help ease the societal burden placed on those who conceive their children in non-traditional ways: through IVF, donation, surrogacy or whatever new technologies are yet to come. I hope the children who come to exist as a result feel normal, loved and accepted by the society they live in. I hope to be the ghostwriter for my own family and other families, shaping our stories into something more positive. Something that's as beautiful and human as anyone else's origin story.

Artificial

Definition

1. Man-made
2. Insincere, contrived
3. Imitation or sham

I asked Mum if she knew who first saw my cells dividing.

'Simon Fishel,' she said.

While Edwards, Steptoe and Purdy had faced a David and Goliath mission when trying to create the first IVF baby, the adversity had not ended there. Simon Fishel worked alongside Robert Edwards at the University of Cambridge as a PhD student, and was part of the core team who set up Bourn Hall in 1980. It was there that he and John Webster treated Lesley Brown for a second time, resulting in Louise's sister, Natalie. When Natalie gave birth to her own child, conceived naturally, in 1999, she was the first IVF baby in the world to have their own baby. Simon and John became the first 'grandfathers of IVF'.

After leaving Bourn Hall in 1984, Simon and John were approached about building an IVF unit in Nottinghamshire, the first of its kind in the Midlands. Before this, Simon had agreed to open a clinic in New York and relocate to the States but decided that Nottingham would be a less disruptive move for his young family. Lucky for me. In 1985, the duo set up the Park Hospital in rural Nottinghamshire, where my siblings and I were conceived. The clinic – nestled in historic Sherwood Forest – was just a few hundred metres from my local bus stop, where my siblings and I caught the bus to school every day. After originally signing up to a long waiting list at a clinic in London, John and Sandra knew they were lucky to have the Park open so locally, and were among the very first patients.

In 1997, Simon founded CARE Fertility, now the largest chain of private fertility clinics in the UK. I learned that Simon had written a book called *Breakthrough Babies* about his pioneering work. I read it and found myself gasping at almost every page; his stories were staggering. While Simon has contributed an immense amount to the world of fertility treatment over the last four decades and achieved a great deal of success, it has come at a cost. Each chapter was brimming with red tape, hostility and lawsuits. Once, a gun was held to his head. Fertility treatment in the 1980s and 1990s, it seemed, had been, quite literally, the wild west.

I emailed Simon to ask if he'd be open to having a chat. I explained that I was one of the many children he'd helped to create and was exploring the history of IVF and donor conception for my own book. He agreed and we set up a video call.

I messaged Mum:

> I'm interviewing Simon Fishel. Do you have any questions?
>
> I didn't have any questions then and I don't have any now. Was happy to be in their hands. Was a wise decision.

A few days later, Simon and his wide smile popped up on my laptop screen. He was sitting in front of a green wall with a framed photograph of a male lion behind him.

'What I've learnt from my work,' he said, 'is that it touches every aspect of humanity: law, ethics, philosophy, politics, medicine, science. If all of a sudden we woke up and everybody on the planet was infertile, what would be the number one political agenda? Because what's the point in carrying on? Why should we worry about climate change? Why should we worry about the economy? Because we're just going to die out within a generation. It becomes vital.'

In his early seventies and despite having semi-retired from the world of IVF, Simon seemed to be bursting with the same passion for fertility treatment he'd had when it was in its infancy.

'So why wouldn't that be just as critical to a couple, to an individual, than it would be to a nation? Because they feel it just as much.'

Simon has many claims to fertility fame, having developed new embryo incubation, chromosome screening and time-lapse technology, all of which improved IVF success rates. In 1987 the World Health Organisation invited him to introduce IVF techniques to China and he has trained doctors all over the world. But his most significant achievement, I believe, was his pioneering work on sperm microinjection. While scientists had made strides in overcoming female infertility by the 1980s – bypassing the fallopian tubes and fertilising eggs outside the body – they had barely addressed issues with sperm.

Simon noticed that when he retrieved eggs from a woman and placed them in a Petri dish with her partner's sperm, sometimes none would fertilise, leaving the couple heartbroken. Some sperm, he realised, were not capable of penetrating an egg. 'This was ground-breaking,' he wrote in his memoir. 'Until then infertility had been considered a purely female issue, but we showed there was more to it than that.'

Could he give the sperm a helping hand, he wondered, by pushing it between the inner layer of the egg and the outer shell? The tools to perform such fine movements at such a minute level, however, did not exist. He needed a more powerful microscope, a very sharp needle – twelve times thinner than a strand of human hair – and something to hold the egg in place.

'The whole concept of trying to pick up a single sperm, which is 150 times smaller than an egg, which is 10 times smaller than a full stop, and shove it into an egg was incredible.'

His colleague found a company run by electronic engineers and tasked them with designing tools for the job, ultimately enabling him to invent a technique called sub-zonal insemination, or SUZI. By 1987, Simon could finally offer SUZI to real patients: 'desperate couples who had no one else to turn to, their only other option being to use donor sperm'.

My older brother, Tim, was born in 1986, too early for SUZI, but why, if my parents were Simon's patients, had they not been offered it for their subsequent rounds of IVF?

'They wouldn't allow it in this country,' Simon said. 'It was the same old scenario.'

The licensing authority in Britain had insisted that he prove the technique was safe – not liable to birth defects – before they would let him practise it.

'Talk about a catch-22: how could I prove it was safe before I used it?'

It was the same dilemma that Robert Edwards had come up against when trying to get funding for IVF. A frustrated Simon was soon invited to set up a clinic in Italy – where there were fewer restrictions – and seized his chance.

In 1990, he welcomed the world's first child born as a result of SUZI, Maria Rosso, a healthy baby girl.

'My clinic in Rome was a stone's throw from the Vatican,' he said, 'and 85 per cent of the women I treated were Catholic. They told themselves that God would want them to have a child.'

By August 1991, the HFEA had been set up in the UK but since it wasn't yet ready to formally inspect IVF clinics, Simon took advantage of a brief opportunity to attempt new technologies like sperm microinjection without restriction. The first British SUZI baby arrived in September 1992. I was born in June 1991. My parents had been fifteen months too early. Had overzealous health and safety regulations prevented them from having full-biological children?

The next time I saw Mum I brought it up.

'Did you know about sperm microinjection?' I asked.

'Yes, but it wasn't around when Tim was conceived,' she replied. 'I'd heard about it when I was back in hospital for you, though.'

'Was it available?'

'I knew they were working on it. I could have asked them and maybe pushed to get it.'

'So why didn't you?'

'I had a conversation with Dad about it. I said, "Do you want me to ask about this new sperm injection thing?" And he said, "No."'

'Why?' I asked, confused.

'He said he was really happy with Tim, so thought we should just do the same again.'

I was moved to hear this.

'But I'm not sure it would have worked,' she continued. 'I think in Dad's case it would have been unlikely.'

'But there could have been a chance,' I said.

Back then SUZI had only a 25 per cent success rate, however everything changed when an Italian doctor in Belgium slipped while performing the procedure, accidentally inserting the sperm into the centre of the egg instead of between the membrane and shell. But rather than cause the egg to leak and fertilisation to fail, as he predicted, it proved to be a very fruitful way of fertilising the egg. His success rate jumped to 70 per cent and he called his technique intracytoplasmic sperm injection, or ICSI. ICSI soon overtook SUZI as the mainstream form of sperm microinjection and today it is performed in two-thirds of IVF procedures around the world. Many clinics in the United States use it as standard for all of their patients.

According to Simon, ICSI has 'allowed 95 per cent of men with sperm problems presenting for treatment to become genetic fathers, even if those problems were extreme'. He described it as a 'revolution'. We'll never know if it might have made the difference for my parents.

The routine 'plan B' route of using donor sperm for couples with male infertility seems to have been a snapshot in time for the history of fertility treatment. In those years between 1978 and 1992 when IVF was available but sperm microinjection was not, patients like John and Sandra were given two choices: half-biological children with a sperm donor or no biological children at all. They chose us.

In the 1980s, donor-conceived children were nothing new. Long before artificial intelligence, AI stood for something else: artificial insemination. We might think of IVF as the first time we separated sexual intercourse from reproduction, but people have been conceived through artificial insemination with sperm donors for more than a hundred years.

In 1884, a thirty-one-year-old Philadelphia woman visited her doctor, William Pancoast, complaining that she was struggling to conceive. After examining her and finding nothing amiss, he examined her husband who admitted he had contracted gonorrhoea in his youth. Microscopic analysis revealed his semen to be 'absolutely void' of sperm, so Pancoast prescribed a course of treatment for the gonorrhoea, but still they could not conceive. Pancoast was at a dead end. Then one of his medical students joked: 'The only solution to this problem is to call in the hired man.' A brilliant idea, Pancoast thought.

Under the guise of a 'medical examination', and surrounded by students sworn to secrecy, Pancoast sedated the woman with chloroform. 'The best-looking member of the class' had agreed to provide a sperm sample and Pancoast injected the fluid into the uterus of the unconscious woman using a hard rubber syringe, then plugged her cervix with gauze. Nine months later, she gave birth to a healthy baby boy.

Later on, Pancoast felt some guilt about the secret and decided to tell the husband, who was delighted, apparently, but conspired with the professor in keeping it a secret from his wife. The details of this story come from a letter to a medical journal written twenty-five years later by one of the medical students who witnessed the insemination.

'It may at first shock the delicate sensibilities of the sentimental who consider that the source of the seed indicates the true father,' he wrote, but, he argued, the origin of the sperm and egg is 'of no more importance than the personality of the finger which pulls the trigger of a gun'.

In other words, the family who raises the child is of more value than the single cells that happened to contribute to its existence.

'Many a man rocks another man's child and thinks he is rocking his own,' he continued. True, though I imagine it is one of very few cases in history in which the father knew the child was not his own while the mother did not.

'I remember a gynaecologist once telling me that he knew a couple of families where the child was delivered at the other end of the street with another family, and quietly handed back,' Simon told me. 'So it was done in their own way. People have done it in their own way since biblical times.'

'Have you heard of a fellow called Derek?' he asked. I had not.

'After World War One many of the men who came home were damaged, and there was no way they could have families. A gynaecologist in London thought it was her mission to help them, so she advertised and eventually found this chap called Derek. Derek would visit the women when their husbands were gardening or away for the weekend or whatever and he ended up producing five hundred children before they retired him.'

These days the service Derek offered would be described as 'natural' insemination, as opposed to 'artificial' insemination, because he had intercourse with the women. A quick internet search reveals that it's still an option offered by some sperm donors today, though by all accounts, not a popular one.

'Then we flip to 2006 when they brought in the ten family rule,' said Simon.

'So when I was conceived in the nineties, did you have any rules on how many families you would use each donor for?' I asked.

'I can't remember how many times it was, but if it was more than five, I'd be surprised,' said Simon. 'We were uncomfortable about using a donor too often.'

I am comforted by this. It must be shocking to find tens or hundreds of half-siblings online, and I am grateful that I can count mine on two hands. Albeit, the ones I know about.

I ask if he ever imagined a world in which donors wouldn't be anonymous any more.

'I thought anonymity would remain anonymity,' he said. 'Of course we didn't even have email, let alone the internet. It was all clinical records. The only way it could happen is if someone somehow managed to break into a facility and find the paperwork with the donor code written on it.'

I had forgotten quite how rudimentary the world was in the early nineties. The internet – the technology Simon and I were using to talk face to face – was not available back then, and it wasn't until the year 2000 that scientists first started to understand the human genome. It must have been unfathomable to medical professionals that, within just one generation, donor-conceived children would be able to upload their DNA sequence to a global system of interconnected computer networks and be matched to their donor.

'Did you have much to do with the recruitment of donors?' I asked.

'We had a person that was specifically doing donation recruitment. We often got it from the donor sperm bank and, if they already had the right characteristics, it could be provided from that, or we'd go on a recruitment campaign. So we were quite lucky that we had a local facility acquiring donor sperm that was already set up decades before us.'

Since 1991, more than seventy thousand donor-conceived children have been born in the UK. Today egg, sperm and embryo donation accounts for 1 in 170 of all births, and for 1 in six IVF births, so it has become relatively commonplace.

'Like most people, I didn't know anything about donor conception before I found out I was conceived that way,' I told Simon. 'These technologies aren't for everyone. Some people will do IVF but never want to do egg or sperm donation, and that's fine. They're just options.'

'Exactly. Some people seem to think that we drag people kicking and screaming into hospitals and force them to have these things, but it's what they want. Our duty is to make it as safe as possible and to provide the information for people to make independent choices.'

I think about all the news articles I've read about new fertility technologies and how often they seem to scaremonger or scandalise. But surely without demand there would be no reason to supply?

'I would love to understand your position or anybody else in your shoes,' Simon said. 'This gossamer thread of genes through families is obviously important, but how important is it to actually being a good parent?'

Gossamer is the fine, delicate silk that spiders use to make their webs. I like the metaphor.

'There is an interesting animal evolutionary model about this,' Simon continued. 'If you've got a lioness with cubs and the father leaves, when a new male comes in, do you know the first thing he does?'

'Kills the cubs?'

'Yes. So, instead, the lioness decides to let him mate with her in the hope that when he sees the cubs, he thinks they're his. And that's exactly what happens, because he doesn't have the intelligence to know that you don't produce cubs in two minutes.' I laughed. 'But actually, he then starts to protect the cubs because he thinks they're his.'

Bringing up another male's children is common in the animal kingdom, whether they know it or not. I'm glad that at least my dad was aware and willing. More than that, he has spent his life encouraging, supporting and loving us as deeply as anyone would their own.

Since retiring from IVF research, Simon has expanded his ambitions into technology that can delay the menopause and potentially prolong fertility. He is also the chair of an advisory board for a company called Genomic Prediction, based in the US, which offers risk-score screening for embryos, a more advanced method of pre-implantation genetic diagnosis (PGD), which is routinely offered today for parents with a known risk of passing on a genetic disorder. He describes them as the first company in the world to offer a 'life view' or health score on embryos; insight into which embryos might have a high potential for certain diseases or conditions.

'Again, it hits real ethical barriers,' he said. 'We all believe in preventive and personalised medicine; I just think people are being empowered with information. You're just trying to avoid illness in children.'

The technology is currently not allowed in the UK and it's obvious why this topic makes some people feel uncomfortable.

For decades critics warned of 'slippery slopes'; that IVF would lead to embryo selection and a kind of eugenics in which children were chosen for certain aspects of their appearance or IQ. For Simon, rubbing up against arguments like these is just part of the process when advances in technology first come about. Throughout his career, treating patients with very specific requirements, he has been accused of being a mad scientist out to create 'Frankenbabies'. He has lived through the controversies of helping to make so-called 'saviour siblings', sister-to-sister egg donation, and the case of a woman who carried her own grandchild because her daughter was unable to.

'When I did the first sister-to-sister insemination,' said Simon, 'I still remember the face of this woman at a meeting in London who just looked at me and viciously said: "You don't know what damage you've just created." But for who, I thought? For the child? For the family? Well, twin boys were born from it and my wife and I were invited to the wedding of one of them a few years ago. They keep in touch all the time.'

The mother of the twins was so grateful she even named one of the boys after Simon. The other she called Robin, after local legend Robin Hood.

Here, Simon mentioned Lesley Brown, mother of Louise and Natalie. 'When they asked Lesley, later in life, what she thought about IVF,' said Simon, 'she said it was wonderful for her and God bless Steptoe and Edwards, but maybe it's going a bit too far now.'

It was hard to know what to make of that. Is technology only going too far when it's something *other people* need?

'She probably thought that anything more might send humanity over an abyss,' said Simon. 'But it was all right for her, because she was just having Louise and Natalie.'

After my conversation with Simon, I abseiled down a rabbit hole of gene theory, trying to understand more about the age-old nature versus nurture debate. It got me thinking: how much do our genes really matter?

'Our fate,' James Watson said, 'is in our genes', but British science writer Philip Ball disagrees. Ball claims that genes are, in fact, not all they've been cracked up to be. Over the last two decades the human genome has been hyped up to be the complete genetic blueprint for human beings; a predetermined instruction manual for each of our lives. But Ball says this is simply not the case.

Claiming we know how genes work, he argues, is like saying that the entire work of Dickens is contained within the dictionary. The words may be there but not in any meaningful order. They are devoid of the unique craft and imagination of a talented writer. Our efforts to unpack our DNA so far, using the four chemical bases of genetic code – A (adenine), C (cytosine), G (guanine) and T (thymine) – are akin to reducing a sentence to the definition of its individual words, or a book to individual sentences. It doesn't really work.

'Each level of the process is not wholly defined by or inherent within the level that precedes it,' Ball writes in his book *How Life Works*. 'To put it another way, what is in that "magic" is something else that the system needs: some added information, context and causal power.' A pen and the alphabet do not a novel make.

When it comes to molecular genetics, humans are yet toddlers, still learning the basics and far from masters of a language that some scientists claim to be fluent in. What's more, Ball argues that genes are simply building blocks, without autonomy or agency. They are servants not masters. In fact, he goes as far as to say that human language is inadequate for describing how these intricate and complex genetic interactions, evolved over millennia, actually work.

What we know is that during embryo selection, if we try to select genes for high intelligence, the probability of distribution means we may indeed improve the likelihood of having a child with a higher IQ – though this is not guaranteed – but we might simultaneously be selecting genes for schizophrenia or neuroticism, for example. In short, nature has a knack of rebelling in unpredictable ways, so we have no real idea what effects our meddling will have in praxis.

'A genome sequence can never "fully specify the organism": how it will grow, how it will look, how it will behave – or in short, how it works,' Ball writes. Genes impart capabilities, he says, but the rest is up to us, in interactions with our environment.

The term coined for this phenomenon is epigenetics. Epigenetics allows us to switch genes on or off, depending on certain lifestyle factors, starting from the womb. Our upbringing, diets, socioeconomic circumstances, stress levels, exercise and exposure to toxins can affect our epigenome and contribute to how our genes express themselves in everything from what diseases we develop to how we age and how susceptible we are to mental illness or substance abuse. Nature and nurture are, in fact, not two separate things but reliant on each other; inextricable.

I found reading Ball's theories about the role of genetics to be somewhat of a tonic. What I have wanted to do for the past six years is to create distance between the donor and myself and to repair the connection between me and my dad. The gossamer thread of our genes is more fragile and irrelevant than previously thought and I found it comforting. A human life is more than the sum of its genes.

The donor may have been the paint, but paint alone does not create art. It needs a canvas on which to come alive. It requires skill and patience and resilience in the face of fallibility. It demands that someone show up to the easel every day and master their tools: brushes, a water pot, time, imagination and, I would argue, most importantly, love. My dad has given us these in reams. The donor has not.

Anonymous

Definition

1. Of unknown authorship or origin
2. Not named or identified
3. Lacking individuality, distinction, or recognisability

In the summer holidays before I started university, Dad asked me to come and work with him for a week to help with an extension he was building for a small twelfth-century church in Lincolnshire. He needed someone to drive a mini-digger. After a few lessons Dad was impressed by how quickly I got the hang of it, so I started to dig a trench ready for water pipes to be installed below ground. One day I came across something hard in the soil. I jumped off the digger and inspected it. It looked like an animal bone. I took it into the church to show Dad.

'We need to stop digging and call the archaeologist,' he said, 'and the vicar.'

'Why?'

'If it's human bones, they'll need to do a report. The archaeologist checks how old the bones are and then the vicar blesses them and reburies them, as a sign of respect.'

For the rest of the day we waited for the archaeologist to arrive. It turned out that I had dug up part of a human hip bone.

As a child, one of my ambitions was to be an educational skeleton. Aged eleven, I remember arriving at my first high school biology lesson and being in awe at the sight of a real skeleton. As I picked up its arms and held its hand, I was mesmerised. When I looked at the bones, it was hard to imagine them as a real person, with a personality, a job and a family. I tried to picture their face and smile, but skeletons do not give much away. We all look pretty similar underneath. This former person would forever be anonymous and unknowable, watching generations of children from the corner of the classroom.

As I grew older, I realised that real human skeletons – their bones scraped of muscle and sterilised, then painstakingly pinned back together for academic display purposes – were not exactly in demand. Most schools didn't have one and any that did had by now likely replaced them with plastic replicas. My dream of being a skeleton in a classroom would probably never be realised, so I decided I wanted my bones to be buried instead.

'I'd love someone to dig up *my* bones one day,' Dad told me that day at the church.

'Me too,' I said, imagining another father-daughter duo unearthing my hip bone in eight hundred years' time.

When I signed up to become an egg donor, one of the requirements was that I give a detailed family medical history on both sides, including grandparents. I realised I would need to ask the donor some questions, but I felt conflicted about contacting him. I believed I had a right to know about my health history – for myself as well as for the egg recipient – yet the act of extracting that information felt like a betrayal of my dad. I wanted Mum's opinion, but she didn't know I was donating my eggs, or that the donor had joined the website. I cornered her one day while she was doing chores.

'Can I talk to you about something?' I asked, helping her change some bedsheets.

'Yes,' she replied. 'What is it?'

'You know . . . the whole sperm donor thing,' I said. She stopped, briefly, and looked at me, before removing a pillowcase.

'Yes.'

'I know we haven't talked about it again.' I paused, my heart pattering. 'But I thought you should know that he recently signed up to the DNA website . . . so I know who he is.'

'What?' She took a step away from the bed, leaving one of the corners loose. 'I wasn't expecting you to say that.' She put one hand on her forehead and stared ahead.

'I know. I was really shocked too.' I gave her a moment to percolate and pulled the sheet over the corner until it was taut. I could see she had a million questions but didn't know whether to ask any of them. Could three decades of anonymity really be reversed? Should it? She looked curious but conflicted. I knew the feeling.

'What did you find out?' she asked finally, then hesitated. 'You don't have to tell me everything.'

'He was a chemistry PhD student at Nottingham University.' I told her his name and age. She looked off into the distance.

'You remember the twins I was in touch with, the half-sisters?' I said. 'Well, they've been in contact with him over email. He seems friendly and has answered all their questions. He said one of the reasons he donated was because he thought that any parents going through the process of IVF would make good parents.' I had hoped Mum would find this comforting, but her expression did not change. She looked deep in thought.

'Are you okay?' I asked.

'Yes, I'm just thinking about how much I want to know.' She paused. 'I don't want to, you know, find out much more than Dad and have to keep it from him.'

'Yeah.'

'Do you have a picture of him?'

'Um, yeah.' As I pulled out my phone and started searching

through the group chat with Libby and Lucy to find the photos the donor had sent, I felt like I was floating away from my body. I had worked out that he was seventeen years younger than Mum and twenty-three years older than me. The same age as her best friend's children; the bumps under her friends' wedding dresses. The missing generation between us. But he wasn't her son, he was the biological father of her children. Of me.

I showed her the photographs and she didn't say much. I had experienced a similar reaction when I first saw them. There were two pictures of him in his twenties, neither of which was particularly clear. One was from a side angle and I could see he had quite a prominent chin, like me, but other than that he just looked like a generic white man with brown hair in a white T-shirt, drinking beer with his friends. He didn't look particularly similar to me or my siblings. His recent photo was more pixelated. Again, a generic middle-aged man with a mildly receding hairline.

'Do you know when he started donating?' Mum asked.

'No,' I replied. 'Why?'

'Well, it's just that I don't know if they used the same donor for Tim or not.'

'Oh,' I said, stunned. 'They didn't tell you if they'd used the same donor or not?'

'No, we just let them get on with it. We didn't ask questions.'

I held back from commenting on how crazy I thought it was not to ask something so important.

'I could ask him,' I said. 'I have his email. But I didn't want to contact him without checking with you first.'

'I'm not going to stop you from doing anything,' she said.

'Okay, thank you. I know it's a bit tricky with Dad. I don't want to bring it up again if it's difficult for him. But I've also decided . . .' I hesitated. 'Well, it's just a bit more complicated because . . .' I was more nervous about this part of the conversation; I didn't want her to react badly.

'I've decided to donate my own eggs,' I continued. 'And they won't let me do it unless I have a full health history from both sets of parents and grandparents.'

Mum's eyes widened and her shoulders dropped forward. She sat down on the unmade bed.

'I haven't told you until now because I didn't know if they'd want my eggs and also because I didn't want anyone to try and change my mind.' I breathed. 'But the counsellor I spoke to – they make you have a counselling session before you do it – said she thought it would be best not to keep it a secret.'

'Right,' said Mum. Everything about her softened: her body, her voice. 'As I said, I'm not going to stop you from doing anything you want to do.'

'Thank you.'

I felt an ache of empathy. It was another hit of unexpected news. First, that the biological father of her children was no longer anonymous, and then, that I was donating her first biological grandchild to a stranger.

A few weeks later, on 1 April 2020, Libby and Lucy set up a group video call with the donor. It may have been April Fools' Day, but as we were ten days into a national lockdown because of a deadly global pandemic, nothing seemed too ridiculous.

As I hid in my room – away from my parents and brother – and plugged in my laptop, I felt a combination of thrill and dread. Since I was spending lockdown with them, we were living in close quarters and ate all our meals together. I had told them I was on a video call with colleagues, so if they heard me talking to unfamiliar voices, they wouldn't suspect anything.

'You were all a lot smaller last time I saw you,' the donor joked when he logged on. 'I was probably holding you in a cup on the bus, rushing to get to the clinic on time.' I shuddered, half-laughing. Another dark sense of humour.

The donor was chatty, confident and articulate, but also a little kooky. He talked about ice ages, death cults and ants being mind-controlled by parasitic fungi. At times it felt like we were sitting in a lecture with an eccentric professor. He told us about the other biological children he knew of: a man called Ben who lived in the south of England, and Russian twins called Eliza and Mike. He said they were all interested in being put in touch.

The call lasted for more than an hour but passed by in a blur, my heart racing throughout as I worried someone would knock on my bedroom door or listen in as they walked down the stairs.

When we logged off, Libby, Lucy and I debriefed over Whats-App, all agreeing how bizarre the experience was and sending each other GIFs of zombie ants.

Within a few days the donor had connected us with Ben and Eliza and set up another group video meeting. I knew this call would last longer and I felt bad spending another evening away from my family, and lying about it. This time they were having a BBQ outside in the unseasonably warm April weather, so at least they were mostly out of the house.

Eliza's brother had decided not to join the call, so it was the donor, Libby, Lucy, Eliza, Ben and me. To my surprise, Eliza spoke perfect English. We took it in turns to tell our stories.

Libby and Lucy's mum had ovarian cysts and their dad suffered with polio as a child, which affected his sperm. They were conceived on their parents' third attempt at IVF. Ben's story was more wacky. His mum and the man he knew as dad, Paul, divorced when he was four years old. During proceedings he was believed by Ben's family to have died of a medical condition and Ben's mum told Ben he was a donor baby, but he hadn't believed it, thinking she was just sparing him the pain of losing his dad. In reality, Paul was actually alive and well elsewhere in the country and years later Ben found him on Facebook. He sent him a message: 'I think you might be my dad.' But Paul explained he couldn't, physiologically, be Ben's biological father following a cycling accident when he was a teenager.

Ben had been conceived by artificial insemination with a donor, after his mother and Paul were selected to trial a new method akin to a turkey baster. On confirmation of the truth, Ben had gone down the official route of contacting the donor through the HFEA, and, because the donor had agreed to be contactable, they were put in touch.

Eliza and Mike had also contacted the HFEA and been connected that way, after their mother had unexpectedly revealed, when they were eighteen years old, that she'd used a sperm donor to conceive them.

I told them my story and how I'd decided not to tell my siblings. Everyone was understanding and seemed to empathise, which made me feel better. When the call ended, I was relieved. I closed my laptop and strode downstairs to join my family outside. It was interesting to meet more half-siblings, but I was struggling to take it all in and felt guilty hiding it from my family. I didn't want any more secrets, but I didn't know what else to do. I filed it away in the back of my mind and helped Mum make a salad.

When the sperm donor signed up in the late 1980s, he was promised lifelong anonymity. Any resulting children, he was told, would never be able to find out who he was. They kept no records. He was unknown, untraceable, genealogically off-grid.

Since he had voluntarily relinquished his anonymity several years ago, I now know the identity of the donor, but for the purposes of this book he has chosen to be identified by a pseudonym: Rodney.

I find this name choice funny for several reasons. When I was growing up, my family used to watch the TV series *Only Fools and*

Horses on repeat. The 1980s sitcom centres around two brothers called Derek and Rodney Trotter, who sell dodgy wares at a market in south-east London. Incidentally, in a later episode, Rodney turns out to be Del Boy's half-brother when he discovers that they do not share the same biological father.

But the donor did not choose the pseudonym because of Rodney Trotter. He chose it from the lyrics of a 1979 song called 'Duchess' by the English rock band the Stranglers. Coming up with an alias from an obscure song about a deluded heiress who claims royal heritage is exactly what I have come to expect from Rodney. We have exchanged several emails a year since I first got in contact and each time he signs off with a link to a music video, or five. He has an unusual sense of humour, a penchant for conspiracy theories and a habit of bringing every conversation back, somehow, to parasitic fungi and mind-controlled ants.

In my first email to him, I asked when he started donating, to try and decipher if he had also been the donor for my older brother. He replied that my brother would have a different biological father because his donations began some time after Tim was born. 'Most of the donors would have been medical students,' said Rodney. 'A few years later a group of us from the chemistry department started donating too. In the month Tim was born, I had just started at the University of Nottingham . . . with Katrina and the Waves starring at the end of freshers' week.'

I felt sad reading his email. It turned out that Tim was a half-sibling too.

Although I had found out more about my genetic health on Rodney's side since contacting him, there was still lots I didn't know about the circumstances that led him to donate and why he chose to relinquish his anonymity. As a journalist, I thought it would be remiss to pass up the opportunity to interview my own sperm donor, so I emailed and asked if he would be happy to answer a few questions over video call for a book I was writing. He agreed.

My first question was why. Why does a young man choose to donate his sperm to strangers?

'I thought that helping others and getting paid for it was pretty cool,' he said.

He'd heard about sperm donation through a friend who knew some other students that were already doing it. Rodney became part of a group of regular donors who called themselves 'Frank's Wank Bank', while others were what he called 'loner donors'. I cringed.

'Do you remember how much you got paid?' I asked.

'It was a tenner, which was a lot then. If I went to the right bar, I could get twenty pints for that.'

While T.S. Eliot measured out his life with coffee spoons, it appears that mine was measured out with lager pints.

'And did you?'

'Sometimes, yeah.'

'Not good for the sperm, though, is it?' I joked, mildly concerned at being the product of alcoholic student culture.

'No, but we did a lot of sport. I could go out all night and then play sports the next day. Football, hockey, cricket, running, aerobics. I did everything.'

'How often did you donate?'

'Two to three times a week for around four or five years,' he replied. 'So that's at least a few litres of sperm.'

I cringed again, wishing I hadn't asked. He explained that they could produce the sample on site in a designated room or at home, but they needed to get it to the lab within an hour. He said he would usually do it at home and get a taxi or bus.

'If the bus broke down we'd have to leg it.' There was more jeopardy to my conception than I had imagined.

Knowing I worked in the television industry, Rodney had

emailed me before the call with an idea for a TV show about sperm donors. He called it 'Spunks' and sent the first few scenes he'd written, complete with a carefully chosen eighties soundtrack. He told me that 'spunks' was what Aussies and Kiwis called 'cute young guys', so it had a double meaning. The mayhem and mishaps of each episode included running out of specimen jars and having to produce samples in dirty public toilets when the medical room was accidentally double-booked. It was disturbing and kind of hilarious to read. I dared not ask how much of it was fiction and how much was fact.

'Did you ever think about any future children born from your donations?'

'Of course. Parallel universes. I had some scary dreams about it. But if anyone was prepared to go through the process of IVF to have children then I thought it's likely that their children would be wanted and loved throughout their lifetime.'

I asked about limits regarding the number of children produced per donor. Rodney said there was an understanding that they wouldn't go above a certain number, although he didn't know the figure. At one point a 'raised eyebrow' at the clinic suggested he may have reached that tentative limit, he said.

'If you'd have been given the option to be anonymous or not back then, what would you have chosen?'

'I would have chosen to be anonymous,' he said. 'Without guaranteed anonymity I probably wouldn't have donated. Although I may have considered it if the "expense money" was considerably more, I don't know.'

At the time Rodney donated, sperm donors had no other option but to be anonymous. He could never find out anything about the parents or the children born, and the families would never know anything about Rodney, beyond the basics of height, hair colour, eye colour and profession; what the HFEA calls 'non-identifying information'. Official recordkeeping only began with the establishment of the HFEA in August 1991, two months after I was born. Before then the creation and storage of human embryos had been neither licensed nor regulated and records were not routinely kept.

In 2005 the UK law changed, removing lifelong anonymity for donors. Anyone conceived from a donation made after April 2005 now has a right to identifiable information about their donor when they turn eighteen. But since only a small number of pre-2005 donors have re-registered as identifiable with the HFEA, it's a rare thing to be directly connected with your donor. If Rodney had not voluntarily signed up to 23andMe or the HFEA database, it's likely that I would never know who he was.

I asked what made him come forward.

'I've seen lots of things on TV and what effect it can have on people. I don't think it's fair not to know where you come from, to be honest, now that I've done it. I saw that some people were very lost. You kind of mature and your attitude changes.'

I asked Rodney if he would encourage others to donate. He said it was a personal choice and wouldn't discourage anyone from doing it as studies showed that most donor-conceived children were fine. But when I told him I was planning to donate my eggs, he advised against it.

'I'll be honest with you,' he wrote. 'From experience, I would avoid all unnecessary medical procedures. It is a well-meaning and thoughtful thing to donate eggs but there are risks . . .'

As well as donating sperm while at university, Rodney took part in a medical trial during which he believes a dirty endoscope was used. Soon after the trial he fell ill – enduring a cytokine storm, vomiting and pelvic pain – the effects of which lasted for years. Thus he was wary of egg donation, being far more invasive than sperm donation. Nonetheless, Rodney still provided me with the information I needed to progress with my egg donation, for which I was grateful. When I mentioned that I suffered with endometriosis, like my mum, he told me he'd recently discovered that his aunt had suffered with it too.

'It means you most likely have a genetic susceptibility to endometriosis,' he wrote. 'Specific DNA mutations matched and inherited from your mother and me.'

I got it from both sides then, I realised.

I asked if the process of donating had changed his view on life.

'I'm a chemist, so it's kind of a synthetic world. Without chemistry it's like magic otherwise. But I also sort of see lots of different sides of me and it's nice to see that a lot of these sides are being fulfilled in different ways by people. I suppose in a strange sort of way, it has brought a little bit more contentment to my life.'

'Tell me about that.'

'I've achieved lots now,' he laughed. 'Just by doing that thing. Nothing much.'

'It's funny,' I said. 'Because it was such a small act that has created all these families.'

'I know. Incredible. But I also know about probabilities. I mean, the probability that you have any life or anyone has any life is as close to zero as you can get. I always think throughout history, you know, there was probably a plesiosaurus out there that was going to eat a little reptilian type thing, but luckily this little thing managed to escape and if it hadn't done that, we wouldn't be here. And that's like everything that's happened in history. Everything is so beyond belief.'

Since the day he connected with us online, Rodney has been generous with his time and answered any questions my half-siblings and I have had. He has shown an interest in our lives and emails to wish us Happy Birthday and Merry Christmas. I am grateful for his openness; I know not every donor-conceived person is so lucky. But at the same time I find myself noticeably agitated when his messages arrive in my inbox. I am glad to know his identity and also quietly furious that he exists. I feel like my life has been trespassed on. One day, out of the blue, a middle-aged man knocked on my door and put a stake in the ground that read 'father'. But that's not what he is. I already have a father, I don't need another one.

Many people imagine the scenario of the donor child desperately seeking out their long-lost parent and trying to establish a relationship, but that's not at all how it's felt for me. For my half-siblings – who are estranged from their dads or bereaved – Rodney's presence in their lives might feel different. Two of them have even met him for a pint, but I know that will never be me.

During our early emails, Rodney mentioned how 'proud' he was and how he could see a little of himself in all of us. It was a nice sentiment, but it made my stomach turn. He has not been responsible for anything that any of us have achieved in our lives and yet here he was, revelling in pride at the accomplished and well-rounded adults we had become. He played no part in our education, maturation or discipline. He didn't change a single nappy or sacrifice anything to look after us. He didn't save up for birthday presents or deal with tantrums or wipe away our tears. So many men do the bare minimum in raising their children and still feel they have a claim to their time or success later on. A sperm donor is the epitome of this; they could not be any more absent from their child's life.

But that's what was agreed, I remind myself. It's what everyone wanted. It's not Rodney's fault. He did a kind and generous thing. Most people don't.

I feel frustrated because I don't know what the rules are; there is no social script for a donor–child relationship. I feel tense when my parents and I tiptoe around the subject, refusing to acknowledge it out loud. It's like he both exists and doesn't; a spectre that will follow me around forever. Rodney's genetic proximity to me feels like a betrayal of my parents, a fissure in my identity. I begrudge all this while also feeling grateful for the opportunity to exist. I know my parents must be grateful too, even if they don't know how to show it.

Rodney donated because he wanted to help people. Yes, he got paid to do it, but so did I. The money was for the inconvenience, but it doesn't replace the altruism. His donation – and mine in turn, directly inspired by his – has allowed some families to have hope and, for the lucky ones, to wake up each morning and watch their children grow.

'The gift of life is the ultimate thing that you can give,' Rodney told me, and I agree.

Egg

Definition

1. An oval object produced by certain female animals
2. A cell produced in the body; ovum

The egg, or ovum, is the largest cell in the human body; the width of a strand of hair and visible to the naked eye. Sperm, on the other hand, are the smallest cells in the body; microscopic but mighty in number. More sperm cells are released during a single ejaculation than the number of eggs a woman has during her entire lifetime.

The female body starts making eggs nine weeks after conception – not birth, conception – while the male body begins producing sperm cells during puberty. While sperm are dying and renewing every day, a woman carries the same eggs throughout her life, their number gradually reducing as she ages.

When it comes to fertilisation – egg meeting sperm – the story tends to follow the same trajectory. The sperm embarks on a treacherous journey through the vagina, cervix and fallopian tube and only the strongest, fastest and most athletic survive. Meanwhile the egg waits patiently, passively, devoid of autonomy. Eventually a single sperm manages to penetrate the tough walls of the egg and fertilises it.

In 1992, anthropologist Emily Martin argued that the narrative most commonly constructed in medical textbooks about fertilisation was based on patriarchal gender roles and stereotypes, 'hidden within the scientific language of biology'.

Twenty years later, Professor Pamela Hill Nettleton found that not much had changed. Building on Martin's theories, she brought them into the twenty-first century by analysing thirty-two YouTube videos about conception. In these she found that sperm were represented 'as little men and embodiments of hegemonic masculinity, with heroic sperm winning the egg prize after a competitive athletic contest fraught with peril', while eggs were portrayed as 'featureless planets floating in a murky void . . . without agency or action'. At their worst, Nettleton argued, the videos echoed 'violent sex, rape, or colonization, with the sperm attacking the egg' and 'male rage at women' depicted as 'inherent at the cellular level'. This persistent gendered narrative, she explained, does not 'coalesce with emerging scientific narratives', which tell a very different story.

Modern scientific theory proposes that during ovulation the follicle containing the mature egg swells until it bursts and ejects the egg. The egg is then directed by the funnel-shaped mouth of the fallopian tube where it is wafted down with the help of cilia – hair-like structures – that propel the egg from the ovary towards the uterus. In the meantime the sperm make their way towards it, assisted by contractions of the uterine walls and fluid released in the fallopian tubes that help them swim better. The egg and sperm work a bit like magnets, with the egg releasing a chemical that the sperm has a receptor for, guiding them in the right direction. When a sperm burrows through the outer shell of an egg, the sperm plasma fuses with the egg's membrane and their nuclei merge into one. The process is far more egalitarian than we have been led to believe. New research has also shown that eggs are selective in which sperm they choose and a woman's egg does not always prefer their partner's sperm.

A few months before I turned thirty, I signed paperwork to agree for my eggs to be fertilised with the sperm of a man I didn't know. Almost a year after I'd first contacted the egg donation agency, the time had come to retrieve my eggs.

I had been sent boxes of medication and instructed how to inject my belly twice a day. After ten days of injections, James and I walked through the doors of the impressive glass-fronted building of the Fetal Medicine Research Institute in south London. We took the lift to the first floor – as I had done many times in the weeks before for ultrasound appointments, assessing how my ovaries were responding – but this time James came with me. Due to the sedation, I was told I would need accompanying home afterwards.

We sat in the large open-plan waiting room. When my name was called I took a deep breath and followed the nurse into the surgical area.

'Is that your partner?' she asked.

'Yes, should he just wait over there?'

'Has he done his sample yet?'

'Oh,' I replied. 'I'm an egg donor, so he's not . . . we're not—'

'Oh, right,' she said. 'Yes, he can stay there and we'll come and get him later. Follow me and we'll get you into your gown.'

I suddenly realised that everyone else that day was likely going through IVF as a couple. They would be led to the operating room while their partner provided a fresh sperm sample, ready to fertilise the eggs. But not us. I felt a pang of sadness.

I put on the hospital gown and was wheeled into the surgery room and sedated through a cannula in my wrist. Twenty minutes later, I woke up in a different room. I noticed the nurse next to me had a necklace shaped like a whale's tail.

'My sister would love that necklace!' I beamed. 'She really likes whales!'

I was giddy and overly chatty, a side effect of the anaesthetic.

Egg

The nurse wheeled me back to my bay, where James was waiting, and I was given tea and biscuits. We had a few hours to wait before they let us leave so I decided to message Mum. In the months since I'd told her about donating she had been supportive and asked for regular updates.

I took a selfie with James leaning over me, his mask around his chin; both of us smiling. Proud parents not-to-be. I sent it to Mum.

> All went well?

In recovery room eating biscuits. They said it went well, 10 eggs collected

> WOW. Super well done!
>
> Do you get to know what happens from here?

Yeah I think they tell me if there's a successful pregnancy and birth

> 10 potential embryos! Possibility of twins!
> You're a superstar.

It was an amazing feeling, potentially helping someone to have a much-wanted child, but it felt even better reading Mum's messages. She sounded so proud.

I thought it would also be a good time to tell my sister, Ruth. I hadn't mentioned anything to her about being an egg donor because I was worried about accidentally blurting out something about our conception. I figured that texting her now would be not only a contained and safe way of telling her, but also some light entertainment. Ruth has always been a worrier, so I thought it would be funny to send her a photo of me in a hospital bed without any context.

> Are you ok??? What's happening???

Lol it's okay. I'm just being facetious. Nothing to worry about, all planned.

> What do you mean?

Last year, during first lockdown, I wanted to do a good deed so I signed up to be an egg donor and today it finally happened.

> Awww that's so lovely

As I know there's a shortage, and have a friend who's been having fertility problems

> Well done Bex. A really great deed indeed. My friend did the same thing a few years ago when she donated eggs as part of a study on mitochondrial DNA.

Ruth told me that her friend from university, Roisin, had a brother who died when he was sixteen. He had inherited a rare genetic disease called Joubert syndrome, causing him to be wheelchair bound and fully dependent on his family. Five years after he passed away, Roisin saw an advert asking for egg donors for research to help prevent genetic disorders. She signed up, wanting to help other families avoid the same devastating loss that her family had been through.

Ruth sent me a link to the study. It was a new IVF technique in which the nuclear DNA from a fertilised egg was transplanted into a donated egg that has had its nucleus removed. Kind of like giving a snail a new shell. The aim was to use the technology to help women with mitochondrial disease avoid passing it on to their children. Families with mitochondrial diseases are few, but the impact can be dreadful. Women who carry such DNA mutations can suffer recurrent miscarriages and many infants do not survive beyond early childhood. But when the first baby was born from this pioneering technology, the story provoked clickbait headlines such as: 'Three-parent baby' and 'Baby with DNA from three people'.

Technically the babies do share DNA from three different people, but the mitochondria forms a minuscule amount, just 0.1 per cent. The donor is not a 'third parent' – their DNA is just a dash of pepper in the soup – though of course, ambiguous headlines like these inevitably incite a potent public response and there are always unkind people in the comments. It was another example of how the anti-IVF rhetoric my parents came up against thirty years ago is still very much alive and kicking today.

A couple of weeks after the egg collection, the agency forwarded me a handwritten letter from the recipient.

Hello dear donor,

I wanted to write to you to thank you from the bottom of my heart for donating your eggs recently for me! I find it hard to express how immensely grateful I am. I know from my experience of IVF over the last few years what an arduous process it is, and I'm frankly really moved that you have done it for someone else. And that lucky someone else is me.

It's an extraordinary thing and although I have not met you, when I read your forms I could see immediately that you were a kind, clever and special person.

Anyway. That's all for now, but again thank you – you have given me hope that one day I might be a mum – and that hope is something I had run out of. You've also taught me a lot about kindness.

All the very best to you.

I cried reading it. It felt so special to see her handwriting and words addressed directly to me. I had been wondering about who she was, what kind of person she might be, and now I knew. She had a beautiful heart, and that's all that mattered. My eggs were a gift from stranger to stranger and now it felt like we were tethered in the cosmos. I would probably never meet her, never know who she was, but I was rooting for her.

Two months later, I was filming a vicar giving birth at home for the BBC midwife series when I received a text message from the agency. My recipient was pregnant. I felt a rush of adrenaline as my mind spun through emotions like a dice, not knowing which it would land on. Joy? Relief? Envy? How are you supposed to react when someone else is pregnant with your biological child?

My colleague Rachel and I were sitting on some steps outside the vicar's house, overlooked by the beautiful Victorian Gothic church where her parish gathered every week. Three hours into the labour, we were giving her some privacy but could hear the howls of childbirth from outside.

'I donated my eggs to someone a few months ago,' I told Rachel. 'And I just found out she's pregnant.'

'Oh my goodness,' Rachel said. 'What a fantastic thing to do for someone.'

After that, I didn't hear anything. A year later I contacted the agency but was told they had no news about my recipient and it was their policy not to contact them. If the recipient wanted to share any further news, that was their decision. I could only hope that she was too busy juggling life with a newborn that she hadn't had time to update the agency.

Immaculate

Definition

1. Perfectly clean or tidy
2. Flawless
3. Morally pure; free from sin or corruption

When I told friends about donating my eggs, most were supportive. They thought it a kind, generous thing to do. But one friend, Natalie, reacted badly.

'Oh my gosh,' she said. 'How could you do that?' It was not the reaction I was expecting. 'Is it too late to get them back?' she asked, panic rising in her voice. I was stunned into silence.

I had known Natalie for more than ten years and she had always been encouraging of my, often quirky, endeavours. This one was no different, I thought, she'll be proud of me.

'Yes, it's all done,' I said. 'I can't get them back. I don't want to.'

'But they are your children!'

'Hold on,' I said, calmly. 'If I tell you why I did it, you might understand.'

I realised that as a mother of three, Natalie could not comprehend this scenario for herself; her children being anywhere else but with her. Eggs were sacred and not to be shared like clothes at a swap shop.

It felt wrong to tell Natalie about my family secret when my own siblings didn't know, but I couldn't bear her negative reaction to my news. It wasn't that I was giving my child away, I explained,

I was just helping another family to have a child they deeply wanted. Like someone did for my family. Her body language changed instantly. She listened and nodded. Her prejudices, like mine, were shifting shape.

But I knew there was another reason Natalie had such strong views. She is a Christian. Her faith is deeply important and forms a large part of her life. I've always been agnostic, and pretty open-minded, so when we were at university I occasionally went along to church with her. One time she introduced me to the pastor, a man in his forties with shoulder-length hair.

'It's lovely to meet you,' he said.

'You too,' I replied. 'I enjoyed your sermon.'

Natalie explained a bit about how she knew me and we chatted for a few minutes. He asked if he could pray for me and, a little bemused, I said yes. We bowed our heads.

'I get the sense that you're like an egg,' he said afterwards. 'Soft and gooey on the inside, but with a hard shell on the outside. You have this tough exterior, but inside you're more fragile.'

'That sounds about right,' I replied, a lump forming in my throat.

When I first discovered that my siblings and I were conceived by IVF, I would tell people, jokingly, that we were immaculately conceived, because our parents didn't have sex to make us. But later on I discovered that I was misusing the term. I thought immaculate conception meant that because Mary was a virgin, she did not have sexual intercourse in order to conceive Jesus. His conception, therefore, was pure, clean: 'immaculate'. But I was wrong. It refers to the conception of Mary herself and the notion that she was free of Original Sin.

I delved further and was surprised to learn that the Virgin Mary's parents, Anne and Joachim, suffered from infertility. In *The Protoevangelium of James*, Joachim was apparently so 'exceedingly grieved' at being unable to conceive a child that he took himself off to the desert for forty days and nights, refusing food or water. Meanwhile Anne began mourning both her husband and her lack of children, until her handmaid had a firm word with her: 'How long do you humiliate your soul?' she said, imploring Anne to just let God do his work.

Nine months later, Anne gave birth to Mary. As a girl, Mary was consecrated to the temple and when she hit adolescence the high priest requested she marry a local widower. Cue Joseph, a carpenter, with six children from his previous marriage who would become Jesus' step-siblings, or half-siblings, depending on how you look at it.

Anne and Joachim's struggle to conceive is a theme that arises throughout the Bible. In the Old Testament there is a long line of bereft, childless couples. The first is Sarah, married to Abraham. In the book of Genesis, Sarah is described as 'barren' and after many years of trying to conceive, she asks her handmaid, Hagar, to have sex with her husband instead. Today we would call this a 'partial surrogacy': a surrogate's egg and womb, with her husband's sperm. When Hagar becomes pregnant, she gloats about her ability to conceive, angering Sarah who banishes her to the wilderness. Many years later, God promises Abraham another son, this time with Sarah, who by then is well beyond child-bearing age. But God explains that nothing is too difficult for him and she soon gives birth to a son called Isaac.

When Isaac grows up he marries Rebecca, but after twenty years of marriage, they do not conceive either. Isaac prays to God who proclaims that 'two nations' are already in her womb, Jacob and Esau. Again the pattern continues with Jacob. Jacob wants to marry a woman called Rachel, but Rachel's father insists he wed her older sister, Leah, first. Ultimately he marries them both, but loves only Rachel.

'When the Lord saw that Leah was not loved,' the scripture reads, 'he enabled her to conceive, but Rachel remained childless.' Leah gives birth to four sons, and hopes this will make Jacob love her, but he doesn't. Wildly envious, and still not pregnant, Rachel reaches a point of despair, shouting dramatically: 'Give me children, or else I die!'

Eventually, Rachel offers up her handmaid, Bilhah, to Jacob, hoping to raise any children they conceive. Bilhah gives birth to two sons, and when Leah sees this she also offers up *her* handmaid, Zilpah.

That's a lot of polyamory and pregnancies; I can only imagine that everyone was exhausted. Jacob goes on to have another two sons with Zilpah, and two more sons and a daughter with Leah. For Rachel it must have seemed like everyone else in the world was getting pregnant apart from her. But then God swoops in again and eventually 'remembered Rachel'. God listened to her and 'opened her womb. And she conceived and bore a son.'

Rachel's prayers had been answered, but her contentment lasted only a few years. She had a second son, but died during his birth.

Before reading these stories, I had no idea that infertility was such a major motif in the Bible. When God said 'Go forth and multiply', it seems that not everyone could. After Rachel come more stories of infertility: the unnamed mother of Samson, Hannah (mother of Samuel) and Elizabeth (mother of John the Baptist). Although I am not religious, I was comforted to discover that the hardship and distress of those who cannot conceive is recognised. But what to make of these stories? Have faith and keep praying? Don't let age stand in your way? Offer up your handmaid instead?

One interpretation of infertility in the Bible is that the experience of suffering heightens the significance of the children that are eventually born. The women whose pregnancies come about by divine intervention all go on to birth important leaders. Obviously, infertile people do not all go on to give birth to prodigies or presidents, but perhaps there is a message in there about how wanted these children are and the way that is channelled into how they are loved and raised. Either way, it seems that God loves them.

I was also surprised by the huge variety of family dynamics in the Bible: blended families, surrogates, half-siblings, stepchildren and non-biological parents. Which brings me to Jesus, whose own conception has confounded historians for thousands of years.

I didn't know where to start, so I messaged Natalie.

> Who would you say is the biological father of Jesus?
>
> **In short we don't believe Jesus had a biological father, but that he is God incarnate. His mother was Mary and he was fathered by the Holy Spirit. The beginning of John talks about the word (Jesus) becoming flesh and dwelling among us.**
>
> Thank you. I'm thinking about it particularly in the context of Joseph being the legal father / guardian to Jesus but not his biological father.
>
> Which is a bit like my dad – who was also a carpenter!
>
> Obviously I know they are totally different scenarios, but it got me thinking that it's an early example of donor conception or a family created in that kind of way.

She replied with three thumbs up emojis.

Jesus' father was an abstract concept and he was raised by a man who was not his biological father, a bit like a donor-conceived person.

I asked Natalie her thoughts on IVF.

> I think it would be down to each different person, I know Christians who've done IVF and Christians who wouldn't. As a church we would definitely pray for people to conceive but wouldn't tell people not to do IVF.

Natalie told me she had some more thoughts and would send them over email. I was grateful for her insight and started to wonder why I felt the need to justify reproductive technologies through a religious lens. Is it because Christianity forms the foundations of the western world and I want to set the record straight? Or because I'm anticipating a Christian backlash against me for writing this book and preparing to defend myself? Or is it because I seek affirmation that God does love me and that I have a right to exist? I'm not sure.

Natalie's email arrived a few days later, explaining that the overall purpose of the Bible isn't a guide for how to live, like many of us might think. The characters, although they are sometimes painted as heroes for children, show themselves to be sinful too and should not form a blueprint for our own lives.

With regards to Jacob and his wives, Natalie suggested that they are not there to show or recommend possible family set-ups: 'In fact we can see in the story that the two wives and two servants creates a painful situation', and yet 'this is the family that God has chosen to be his people'.

'Ultimately,' she wrote, the topic of infertility in the Bible 'explores the problem of suffering, particularly the inequality and unfairness of suffering – something that raises big questions and that so many believers and non believers struggle with. But often it is in our times of hurt and suffering that we have to look beyond ourselves and seek God. Where the world says we're lacking, God says we're loved.'

Since learning about how I was conceived, I have felt somewhat cornered and threatened by Christianity, but Natalie's words brimmed with compassion and empathy.

'I hope I've expressed the dignity and love that God has for those struggling with fertility,' she continued. 'Of course there are many ways in which this has been misapplied or misused throughout history and sadly nowadays too.'

I had always known that there was a realm in which science and religion could exist peacefully together, which makes it more frustrating to read about religious leaders who have little tolerance, or outright hatred, for the way that my family and others have been conceived. When it comes to creating new life, I believe that science and religion can co-exist. They already do.

'The barren in the Bible would have felt shame at being outcast, but the creator of the world saw them and loved them,' Natalie ended her email. 'People are loved by God regardless of how unconventional their family or their coming into the world may be.'

Despite not being particularly religious, my parents christened their children and chose names from the Bible for all of us: Timothy, Rebecca, Joseph and Ruth.

'I'm writing about the Bible,' I said to Mum a few months ago. 'I didn't realise how much infertility there is in it.'

'Can I tell you my favourite story about God?' she said. I hadn't known her to mention any stories about God, ever, so I was surprised she had a favourite.

'There's a poem called "Footprints", about someone walking along a beach and looking back through her life. She sees two sets of footprints in the sand, one is hers and the other is God's.'

Mum's eyes turned glassy. 'I get emotional even just thinking about it,' she said, her voice trembling.

'And the woman looks back and notices that during all the hardest times of her life there was only one set of footprints and she says to God, "I don't understand, why did you abandon me at the times when I needed you the most?"'

Mum wiped away tears.

'And God said, "No, it was then that I was carrying you."'

Golden

Definition

1. Containing gold or the colour of gold
2. Having talents that promise great success
3. A fiftieth anniversary of a significant event

In 1925, when Frida Kahlo was eighteen years old, she boarded a bus that determined her destiny. A collision with an electric streetcar left several passengers dead and Kahlo with a broken spine, leg and collar bone. Her pelvis was impaled by a handrail, 'like a sword through a bull'. Her medical notes state that the iron pole entered through her left hip, 'exiting through vagina and tearing left lip'.

'I lost my virginity,' she said of the accident. 'A kidney was bruised, I couldn't urinate, but the thing I complained about most was my backbone.'

Despite the horror of the accident, every version of this story I have read infuses it with a dreamlike quality. Kahlo's clothes were torn off during the impact and another passenger was carrying a pouch of powdered gold that billowed over her. When her boyfriend found her, she was lying naked on the road in a pool of her own blood, covered in flecks of gold.

'Gold was sunlight on asphalt. Gold was the gleam of metal through an open wound,' wrote Leslie Jamison in the *Paris Review* about the incident. But was Kahlo really nude, bleeding and covered in gold dust or has the story been pigmented by time – romanticised, sexualised, fetishised – as depictions of women and girls so often are?

What we do know is that when Kahlo arrived at hospital there was a significant delay in her treatment because doctors wanted to focus on patients who they felt had a chance of surviving. Her boyfriend pleaded with them and eventually they agreed to operate, saving Kahlo's life. She spent three months on bed rest at the Red Cross hospital in Mexico City.

Until then Kahlo had wanted to become a doctor herself, but, unable to continue her studies and bored of lying in a full-body cast, she began to paint. Her mother fashioned a canopy with a mirror above her bed so she could use herself as a model and Kahlo became an artist instead.

Frida Kahlo's face has become an emblem of hope and courage, one reprinted and recognised around the world. In the hundred years since the accident, her story has gained almost mythical status. Her art exists because of her agony. She never painted the accident, though she did sketch it once. It is a crude drawing in grey pencil; there is no gold.

Kahlo's art speaks to people because it is authentic and intimate in the most gruesome sense. Often depicting her own face adorned with floral headbands, she also painted herself murdered, dying and in hospital beds after multiple miscarriages. Her life may be remembered like a fable, but she did not paint fairy tales.

A large black-and-white portrait of Frida Kahlo hangs in my living room. Her eyes follow me wherever I stand or sit. Her black hair is cut in a scruffy bob and her iconic eyebrows meet softly in the middle. Kahlo was queer, having relationships with men and women, and playful with gender and clothing; famously wearing her father's suits and emphasising her facial hair in portraits. While I am strongly drawn to her androgyny now, as a teenager I obeyed a more conformist female aesthetic. Dyed blonde hair, make-up, short dresses, heels. It was the 2000s, the era of Britney Spears, Christina Aguilera and Paris Hilton. The first time I kissed a boy, I was dressed as Marilyn Monroe.

When I got to university, I tacked a poster of Monroe on to my bedroom wall. It was part of 'The Ballerina Sitting' portraits by Milton Greene, hailed as one of *TIME* magazine's most iconic photographs of the twentieth century. In the picture Monroe is wearing a white dress with sheer netting covering her from knee to ankle. You can't tell from the angle of the photograph, but the dress is unzipped, having been ordered two sizes too small by accident. Yet Monroe made it work, pinning the bodice to her torso with her arms and posing with ease; artfully holding the dress together. Holding herself together. When I look at this portrait now I am reminded of Frida Kahlo's *The Broken Column*, another white corset, another body dismantled by surgery and reassembled by scar tissue.

Monroe is one of the most admired archetypes of feminine beauty in modern history with her full figure, golden hair, irresistible smile and a sex appeal few have been able to match. She was one of the most photographed women in the world and is still one of the most famous women ever to have lived. But few people know that she suffered from severe endometriosis.

According to her first husband, Monroe's periods were so bad that the pain would 'knock her out' or, if she was driving, cause her to suddenly 'brake her car, jump out and crouch on the ground in agony'. A biographer once counted fourteen boxes of pills in her dressing room, almost all of them painkillers prescribed for menstrual cramps.

The gold standard treatment for endometriosis in the 1950s was surgery to remove the ovaries and uterus, but because Monroe wanted children she refused it. When she was wheeled into the operating theatre at the age of twenty-five to have her appendix removed, the surgeon found a note taped to her abdomen.

> Dear Doctor,
>
> Cut as little as possible. I know it seems vain but that doesn't really enter into it. The fact I'm a woman is important and means much to me. Save please (I can't ask enough) what you can – I'm in your hands. You have children and you must know what it means – please Dr Rabwin – I know somehow you will! Thank you – thank you – thank you. For God's sakes Dear Doctor no ovaries removed – please again do whatever you can to prevent large scars.
>
> Thanking you with all my heart.
> Marilyn Monroe

Her ovaries were left alone, but four years later Monroe endured her first miscarriage. An ectopic pregnancy and three further miscarriages followed. Although endometriosis tissue was found inside her fallopian tubes, it seems that she was able to conceive naturally but unable to carry a child to term. It is thought that endometriosis increases the likelihood of miscarriage due to inflammation, altered immune function, compromised egg quality and distorted anatomy of the pelvis.

I find it moving to realise that Monroe was not only silently struggling with a debilitating illness and recurrent miscarriages that the cameras could not see, but also under constant public scrutiny for their effects on her life. Throughout her career and beyond, nasty rumours spread that she was unreliable, always late to set, difficult to work with and addicted to prescription drugs. She was a relatively private person and while few know about her endometriosis and fertility struggles, perhaps even fewer realise that she was a poet. Monroe regularly jotted down her musings and poetry in notebooks and on scraps of paper in hotel rooms. In 1955 – when she was twenty-nine – she wrote a poem on a hotel notepad that offers an insight into her state of mind. 'You must suffer,' it begins before describing the loss of her 'dark golden' – an oxymoron perhaps – and how she must be alive 'when looking dead'.

Many of us can relate to putting on a mask for the outside world, but being a Hollywood star must exacerbate the difference between how one feels and how one is perceived. Chronic illness and show business don't mix well.

Despite winning the Booker Prize twice and marrying her childhood sweetheart, Dame Hilary Mantel described endometriosis as a 'destroyer of careers, families and relationships'. But how, with such worldwide acclaim and a marriage spanning four decades, can this possibly be true?

'Anything I have achieved,' Mantel wrote, 'has been in the teeth of the disease.'

I think about that statement often. Anything we achieve is in the teeth of the disease. We may romanticise the notion of the suffering artist, but is suffering really a necessary part of art? Does it make our art better, worse, or perhaps just more closely attuned to our humanness? Does spending days on the sofa, in bed or on a hospital ward, humbled by pain, make us better thinkers, listeners and observers? Less likely to take for granted the good days we do get? Or does it just mean that the art exists at all, when the time and space it inhabits would otherwise have been swallowed up by a 'normal' job?

In a radio interview with Mantel in March 2020, BBC broadcaster – and fellow endometriosis comrade – Emma Barnett asked how she managed a life of pain.

'We all hate being up against something that's impossible,' replied Mantel, 'an obstacle that you simply can't negotiate your way around, so you have to dig underneath it in a way, come out the other side into another world, not one you expected but there it is and make the best of it.'

For those of us with conditions like endometriosis, the best we can do is carry on with our lives, bending our careers and lifestyles around the snags and hurdles we come up against along the way. Ideally we find friends and colleagues who accept our bad days and offer to help.

While living in San Francisco in 1930, Frida Kahlo sent a letter to her mother:

'I am writing this with horrible handwriting. I am lying down because as usual I have some inflammation. But the wives of the other artists have treated me very well; one came over and put a hot-water bottle on me and another one swept the floors for me and cleaned the whole house.'

I have written much of this book lying down, with a hot water bottle and TENS device clamped to me like barnacles. On days when my lower back gripes and my belly swirls with burning, lying down, with my laptop propped on a pillow, offers some minor relief. Of course, in a normal office job this would be unthinkable, as would daytime baths or midday naps, however productive I am on my good days. Mantel said her illness narrowed her career options, making a nine-to-five job almost impossible, so she became a writer.

With regards to relationships, Mantel told Barnett that her 'illness and the crises it occasioned' were 'too difficult to surmount', leading to the breakdown of her marriage in her early thirties.

In a 2005 article for *The Times*, she wrote:

Communication broke down and I was in constant pain with endometriosis. We had felt ambivalent about children but after a hysterectomy at 27, I was furious at not having the choice. I had planned for health and success but got illness and failure. There was a power imbalance in our marriage.

They separated, but it wasn't to be the end of their love story. 'After two years apart we had both changed,' she wrote. 'I'd never stopped loving him but walking away helped us to grow up. We were both needy but now we're emotionally self-sufficient. I've learnt to ring a friend, not talk about everything to my long-suffering husband.'

The couple remarried the year after they divorced (coincidentally, Frida Kahlo and Diego Rivera did the same, forty years earlier), but the reality of living with a chronic illness is clearly one of conflict, crisis management and adaptation. I certainly know the strains endometriosis has caused within my own relationships. I know what it is like to be sick of your own broken-record voice: tired, aching and complaining to your partner, all the while pretending to be fine for everyone else. Functioning in the outside world for as long as possible, then collapsing into a heap at home. Your partner is your safety and sanctuary, but they are sick of being left with a husk of the person they love. They wish they could take away your pain, but they can't. It is frustrating for everyone.

Endometriosis brings its ironies. Pregnancy is often touted as a cure, but infertility can be a symptom. Marilyn Monroe was a global sex symbol and yet sex was probably painful. An invisible and less spoken about symptom of endometriosis is dyspareunia – painful intercourse – experienced by two-thirds of women with the condition. Some encounter pain during sex, others experience it afterwards (which can last from a few minutes to a few days) and some find sex too painful to attempt at all without painkillers or careful planning around their cycle. Depending on where the endometriosis is located, some women report that all penetration hurts, while for others it's only deep penetration, certain positions or certain times of the month. Unsurprisingly, this can affect libido for both partners.

I enjoy sex but it has taken time to retrain my brain; teaching my face not to wince when it feels like I'm being stabbed from the inside. No one wants to have sex with someone who is bracing themselves or gritting their teeth. Over time I have learned how to cajole my body's reflexes and override pain with pleasure, but I have had to accept that for me sex will almost always involve some degree of pain. To manage it, I find that a break, a change of pace or position and slowed breathing can help, and I am grateful to have mostly had responsive and understanding partners, though that hasn't always been the case.

TV host, model and author Padma Lakshmi suffered endometriosis symptoms as a teenager that left her bedridden for several days a month. These included headaches, severe cramping, nausea, numbness, lower back pain, digestive issues, moodiness, swelling and bloating. Her symptoms were dismissed or misdiagnosed for over twenty years until she was referred to an endometriosis specialist. As a presenter on reality cooking show *Top Chef*, Lakshmi got through long filming days with a discreet toolkit. 'We used to plug in my heating pad under the judges' table,' she said. 'After the first few seasons, I got a dressing room so I could lie down on a couch.'

Lakshmi would go on to co-found the Endometriosis Foundation of America with her doctor, Tamer Seckin, in an effort to prevent other women from suffering the way she had. 'It locked me out of my own life,' she said. 'It was not my wish to get up in front of a room and talk about my vagina. But I had to step up. I just want young women to know they're not alone.'

I also had no desire to write about such intimate parts of my life, but needs must. If we don't talk about these things we don't know about them, and if we don't know about them we can't get help or raise awareness. Silence is not golden.

In 2004, Lakshmi married the author Salman Rushdie, but the marriage lasted only three years. When they divorced she revealed that he had described her as a 'bad investment' due to her endometriosis.

'It is a reproductive illness which attacks you at a very vulnerable phase in your life and it really mangles and moulds your attitude towards your femininity,' Lakshmi explained. 'It wasn't the only reason, but certainly one of the big reasons why my marriage fell apart.'

Lakshmi wanted children but was told she may never be able to conceive naturally.

Eight months after I donated my eggs, and three years into our relationship, James agreed to start trying for a baby. I was quietly thrilled. But after six months of periods, I began to worry.

Self-blame seeped in and I questioned everything. Was it because we didn't have sex that one day out of ten in a row? Perhaps that spicy curry I ate had scuppered ovulation? Was my face cream causing oxidative stress to my eggs? I kept track of dates and peed on ovulation strips, but the blood on the tissue two weeks later humbled our efforts every time.

Meanwhile many friends appeared to get pregnant with ease, some on their second or third pregnancies, planning their due dates around work or career changes. I know of several couples who only had sex once every six months and were as surprised as anyone to be pregnant. I nodded and smiled and said congratulations.

Two other friends told me about having abortions in their thirties. Both were in long-term relationships and wanting children in the future, but decided it wasn't the right time. I don't know how to feel about these stories; I sympathise, but they sting and leave my mind aching for days.

For women in their early thirties, the chances of conceiving each month are 15–20 per cent, but for people with endometriosis it drops to 2–10 per cent, depending on the severity of the disease.

My parents tried to conceive naturally for fifteen years with no luck. My aunt tried for two decades over two marriages and died childless. My other aunt, however, is now a great-grandma, with four generations of naturally-conceived children.

To her surprise, Padma Lakshmi eventually conceived her daughter naturally, at the age of thirty-nine. Stories like hers give me hope and I am regularly told similar tales by well-meaning friends about people they know who got pregnant after many years of trying. But at what point do you change tack and try something else, I wonder. How long do you wait?

Despite contending with endometriosis and fifteen years of infertility, my parents' marriage has survived. In 2021 they celebrated fifty years together; their golden wedding anniversary. There was no big party or fireworks, just a few picturesque days away to the seaside as they wished, with plenty of good food and sparkling wine, organised and paid for by their children. It's the least we could do.

But for some couples, pain and infertility turn out to be insurmountable. We might sign up for a life shared with one person, but chronic pain can leave us with someone different, affecting our future in ways we did not anticipate. Infertility is a kind of grief; living with it can be a grating cycle of hope and loss, frustration and loneliness. It puts us in determined pursuit of something that might be unattainable. It removes us from ourselves.

Marilyn Monroe was married and divorced three times. In one of her diaries she wrote, 'I am always alone no matter what.' She was one of the most visible women in the world and yet she felt alone. When the cameras cut, when the exhibition is over, when the book launch ends, we do not see inside the despairing mind and the body hijacked by pain. We are not privy to the opportunities, relationships and everyday delights that are gobbled up by illness or the anguish of infertility.

In the early 1960s, as Monroe's divorce from playwright Arthur Miller was being finalised, she was in and out of hospital for depression, endometriosis and sinusitis. She had been filming a movie called *Something's Got to Give*, and in the end it did. Apparently Monroe had been drawn to the role because she got to play a mother, a departure from the parts she was usually offered such as showgirl, mistress or gold digger. But after just three months of filming, she was fired by Twentieth Century Fox for 'spectacular absenteeism' and sued for $750,000 for 'wilful violation of contract'.

Two months later she was dead. Monroe overdosed on prescribed barbiturates. On the inquest paperwork, under 'mode of death' the coroner circled both 'accident' and 'suicide'. Above suicide, he wrote 'probable'.

The day her death was announced to the world, Monroe's friend Marlon Brando recalled that everyone around him 'stopped work, and you could see all that day the same expression on their faces, the same thought: "How can a girl with success, fame, youth, money, beauty . . . how could she kill herself?"'

Frida Kahlo also died in bed next to a bottle of pills. While some believe she died by suicide, her official cause of death was recorded as a pulmonary embolism. Five months earlier she had written in her diary: 'I've had centuries of torture and at moments nearly lost my reason. I keep wanting to commit suicide. Diego is the one who stops me.'

Monroe was just thirty-six when she died, Kahlo just forty-seven. Their legacies may endure as lives tormented by psychological and physical pain, culminating in the tragedy of their deaths, but in remembering them like this we risk neglecting the true life force they emanated.

'It isn't tragedy that governs Frida's work, as has been wrongly believed by many people,' her husband said. 'The darkness of her pain is merely a velvety background for the marvellous light of her biological strength, her superfine sensitivity, shining intelligence, and invincible strength to struggle for just being alive.'

For some people staying alive is a struggle, for others creating life is a struggle, and for some it is both. I love Rivera's image of a person's darkness illuminating their light.

A year ago, during one of the darkest periods of my life, a friend invited me to get a tattoo with her. I ended up getting three: a triangle on my ankle to symbolise my family, and a sun on one arm and a moon on the other, to represent the light and the dark.

Eighteen months after I learned about my conception secret, an advice column called *Dear Sugar* opened up for submissions after a few years' hiatus. I adored the original column written by Cheryl Strayed and listened to every episode of her subsequent podcast (co-hosted with Steve Almond) throughout my twenties. Strayed's personal life had been shaped by poverty, bereavement, divorce and addiction, and her advice was always wise, astute and hard-won. Her writing is beautiful and deeply considered; she is one of those people who makes you feel like an old friend. In short, I would trust her opinion on almost anything.

With few people to turn to about my dilemma, I decided to write a letter to Strayed to ask whether she thought I was making the right decision by keeping the family secret. I explained my situation in the first half of the letter. The second half read:

> So here's my dilemma. I have three siblings. None of them know about the sperm donor. When my parents told me the truth it was a heartbreaking conversation. I had only ever seen my dad

cry once before, when his mum died. So in that moment I wished I hadn't found out. The secret could have been a secret forever, I would never have known. I didn't need to know. We agreed not to tell my siblings for the time being which was a relief for all of us. I couldn't stand the idea of watching my dad's heart break again, and managing his feelings on top of my siblings and my own. I didn't want to have to fix something that wasn't broken in the first place.

We are a close, happy family but my brother has suffered with mental health problems and my dad is 70 and has a heart condition. If either of those were worsened by revealing the news to my siblings, I wouldn't be able to forgive myself. But do they have a right to know about their genetic identity? Does it matter? Is it insane to keep that information from them?

I've been through therapy and made peace with the bombshell news, but it took me a while. And although I feel that my siblings would also come to terms with the news in time too – and I would certainly make sure the news was delivered to them in a less traumatic way than mine was – is it really necessary to trigger them going through all that? If they sign up to the website themselves organically, my parents and I are prepared for it and will sit everyone down, but do I have a duty to tell them anyway? I have no idea how they will react or what pain they may or may not go through. I don't think they will be angry at me for keeping it a secret, but why set off a grenade and hurt everyone's feelings if I don't need to? After all, it was never my secret . . . and yet I am now the reluctant gatekeeper of it.

After eighteen months of thinking, I feel that keeping this secret is the best and kindest thing to do for my siblings and my parents. But I do have doubts sometimes. There aren't many people whose opinions I trust – who know how non-black-and-white the world is, who have lived and soared through its grey clouds of ambiguity like you have, Sugar – do you think this is the right decision?

Yours,
Reluctant Gatekeeper

Unfortunately I did not get a reply. But two years later, one of Sugar's newsletters arrived in my inbox. It was written by an American mother of triplets who were now in their twenties. It explained that she and her husband had become parents through a sperm donor because her husband had been rendered infertile after treatment for testicular cancer. They had decided to keep it a secret that he was not their biological father. I could not believe what I was reading; the story was so similar to my own. The woman who wrote the letter was asking for Sugar's advice about whether to tell her children the truth, particularly since they had expressed interest in signing up to a DNA website to look for distant relatives.

The end of the mother's letter read:

> In the novel 'The Leopard', Giuseppe Tomasi di Lampedusa wrote about the 'golden moments' that come to us when we're at death's door – our happiest memories that have been stamped on our minds. Most of my golden moments were with my precious children. I could not bear to go on if they rejected me because of this revelation.

I knew this anxiety. I also couldn't bear to think about my family being torn apart by such a revelation, even if only temporarily. Why ruffle any feathers? Ignorance is bliss. If it ain't broke, don't fix it. I was clinging on to clichés like life rafts.

Of course, I was desperate to read Sugar's reply. She was remarkably direct in her response.

Dear Anguished Mom,

There's a line in The Leopard you might find useful: 'If we want everything to stay as it is, everything has to change.' It strikes me that where you are at this moment – realizing that for you to continue to be the loving and nurturing mother you so clearly are, you must do it differently than you have before. You need to shift so you can sustain; reverse course so you can move forward.

You're so right that you must tell your children the truth about their genetic origins, Anguished. Even though it will unravel so much about what they've believed to be true about themselves. Even though it will likely cause them to feel sad or angry or confused or all three. Even though it may temporarily increase the sense of loss and devastation they already feel about their beloved father. Even though it will pain you to pain them.

Sugar went on to say that the secret, which very likely began with love, was now twisted into a lie that only the truth could untwist. By telling her children, Sugar explained, the mother would be making the more ethical choice; opting for honesty over deceit and preventing them from learning the truth in a more traumatic way.

You apologise for having lied to them. You tell them what you wish you'd done if you could go back in time and do it differently. You support them as they navigate the emotions this revelation brings up. You keep talking about it whenever they want to. You answer their questions. You offer them resources. You help them hunt down information if they want to seek it. You give them space. You stay open to the various paths they may wish to pursue in relation to finding and connecting with genetic family members.

'You remember the golden moments,' Sugar's letter ended. 'You let them wash over you. You know they were golden for them too.'

Like Kahlo, Monroe and Mantel, my parents' life trajectory had not gone to plan. They wanted children and they could not have them. But they lucked out; they happened to live at the dawn of a golden age of fertility treatment. Unlike the generations before them, they were offered choices and, like the parents in the letter, they grabbed the opportunity with both hands. They were given a few per cent chance, but it worked. They hit the jackpot and we were the prize. Deception was the cost, but together, somehow, we could undo that debt.

You need to shift so you can sustain; reverse course so you can move forward.

Sugar's reply, gilded with gold, had such a profound effect on me. I knew it was a sign that I had to tell my siblings the truth.

Hen

Definition

1. A female bird
2. A fussy middle-aged woman
3. A woman due to be married

'Have you heard of 23andMe?' Mary, Sophie's mum, asked my sister and me, as we waited for our pedicures. It was a few days before Sophie's wedding and we were getting our nails done, excited that one of the wombies was getting married.

'Yes, I did a DNA test with them years ago,' I replied. 'How come?'

'Well, we all signed up as a family at Christmas,' Mary said. 'And we just got the results back. We're 3 per cent Scandinavian. It's all so interesting, isn't it?'

'Mhmm,' I replied, my face getting hot.

'To be honest I was relieved that Sophie, Zoe and Robert are all actually related to their dad. You never know with IVF, I guess!' she laughed.

'Yeah,' I smiled, hoping the conversation would stop.

'What did you find out?' Mary asked.

'Mainly British and Irish, a little Scandinavian too. I have a slightly increased risk of late-onset Alzheimer's, and that's about it,' I said.

'You've got the app on your phone, haven't you?' Ruth chipped in.

'Yeah,' I said, desperately hoping she wouldn't ask me to open it. This would not be an ideal way to find out.

Luckily I was called for my pedicure. Disaster averted. But it felt like a close call, another elephant in the womb. I felt guilty keeping the secret from Ruth, with whom I usually shared everything.

A year later, at Ruth's hen party, I found myself crying on the bathroom floor like a bad cliché. We were staying in a beautiful manor house in the Cheshire countryside and Ruth and I were sharing a room with our sister-in-law, Gina. Just four hours into her hen party, Ruth was vomiting in the toilet, wearing a leopard-print 'Bride' sash drooped around her knees, surrounded by her closest friends. After playing party games around her for a few hours, we eventually carried her upstairs and put her to bed.

I used this as an excuse to go to bed myself. I had been working night shifts on a medical TV series and my body clock was askew. I was tired but excruciatingly awake. I was also feeling sad. James and I were having no luck getting pregnant and it was weighing on my mind.

Earlier in the evening the hens had all been drinking and chatting and, inevitably, the conversation had turned to children. Most of the other women were mothers and the conversation soon steered into how quickly people had fallen pregnant.

'I'd only been off the pill a few days,' said one.

'I got pregnant the first month as well,' said another. 'They tell you to come off the pill early and that it might take time and bam, you're pregnant instantly.'

'Mine took a few months,' said another. 'My second was fast, though.'

'I wasn't even planning mine,' said another.

And so the conversation continued, in what felt like a gathering of the world's most fertile women, and me. I retreated to the kitchen to get some space.

Later in bed, I lay fully awake, plunging into a spiral of worry. I wanted to talk to Ruth but didn't want to wake her. I tiptoed to the bathroom, hoping she wouldn't hear me sobbing.

At 4 a.m. I texted Mum. I assumed she'd be awake because thirty years after having triplets, she still suffers from insomnia.

Are you awake?

Yes

I'm at Ruth's hen do but haven't slept for two days and I'm crying in the bathroom because I'm so frustrated. I don't know what to do.

What's wrong?

I've been working night shifts and only had 2 hours sleep yesterday morning. Also everyone is talking about pregnancy / their kids / how easy it was to get pregnant, and I just keep having to take myself away because it gets me so down.

I just feel really far away from where I'd hoped to be by age 32.

Your life is your own so don't compare it to others.

But it's not about comparing, it's about not having the things I would really like: a house, children, marriage.

And with children I will run out of time, kinda feels like I already have.

Your mum was eight years older than you when you were born don't forget.

Gina walked into the bathroom and was surprised to see me on the floor. I told her why I was struggling to sleep, but since she was a few years younger than me and had a two-year-old daughter, I worried she wouldn't understand.

'We were trying for ages,' she said, 'and then it happened after ten months, when we stopped thinking about it. I know it's hard, but try to relax. Use it as an excuse to go on holiday.'

'We've been on lots of holidays,' I sighed. 'I have endometriosis like Mum, and her tubes were blocked so she physically couldn't get pregnant naturally.'

'But you're not necessarily going to be the same as your mum.'

'I know,' I said. 'Though it is genetic. I'm just feeling overwhelmed.'

We hugged and I felt calmer. By then it was 5.30 a.m. and I had not slept a single minute, but figured it was too late to try. I crept downstairs and wandered around the garden barefoot as the sun rose, drinking a glass of milk.

After a day of hen party activities – puppy yoga and garden games in animal-themed fancy dress – we returned to the house and made use of the hot tub. After a while just Ruth, Sophie and I were left. I told them that James and I were on the list for fertility tests and I was waiting to get my fallopian tubes checked. Sophie told me that both of her sisters-in-law were struggling with infertility too. One had been trying for two years and the other for ten.

'Wow. That's so hard,' I said. 'Does it make you think about when you guys might start trying?'

'Well, we're planning to move to Australia for a year, and do a bit of travelling,' she replied. 'But we have talked about sperm donors and doing fertility treatment when we get back. And I wondered about freezing my eggs in the meantime.'

'I have mixed feelings about egg freezing,' I said. 'The success rates are not as good as people think they are, and it's pretty expensive. Obviously it's better than nothing, but you're probably better off just finding the sperm now and freezing embryos, rather than eggs, as they're much more likely to survive the thawing process.'

Sophie and her wife, Orla, had two male friends they were considering asking to donate their sperm, and we discussed the pros and cons of the child being biologically related to a friend or somebody anonymous. I desperately wanted to tell her about how Ruth and I had been conceived but I couldn't. Instead I changed the subject, to a book I'd just finished reading.

'It's called *A Heart That Works* by Rob Delaney, the American actor, but he lives in London,' I said. 'It's about his son Henry who was diagnosed with a brain tumour just before his first birthday. It made me laugh and cry and truly appreciate the NHS. All the doctors and nurses and play therapists who looked after Henry sound so amazing. He writes about them with such love and admiration.'

I knew Sophie worked at one of the hospitals where Henry was looked after and I wondered if she was one of the nurses who had cared for him. Due to patient confidentiality, she couldn't tell me but all of our eyes welled up as she told us about how she had cared for many children with brain tumours similar to Henry's throughout her career.

I waded over to her side of the tub and hugged her. 'You're so special. I'm so proud of you.'

Eighteen months later, this conversation would come careening back to me, infused with more significance. There would be no trip to Australia and one of us would go on to freeze our eggs, but it wasn't Sophie.

'Imagine you're in a restaurant and you've ordered your meal, but for some reason everyone else's meal has arrived but yours is still not ready. And some people didn't even order anything and their meals have arrived as well. And then the waiter finally comes with your meal, but they trip and it all falls on the floor, so then you have to wait again.'

Aisling, Sophie's sister-in-law, was explaining to me what it feels like to be in the throes of infertility. Over the years we've got to know each other at birthday parties and BBQs, her beaming smile and firm hugs always leaving a warm impression. I was speaking to her over video call on a Friday morning, grateful that she could fit me in around her busy schedule as a consultant in emergency medicine at Croydon University Hospital. I know from filming in A&E departments what a demanding job it is, involving literal life-and-death decisions on a daily basis. I could not imagine dealing with the emotional exhaustion of infertility on top.

'That grief-hope cycle is just torture. Every month you think, this could be it and it's not. And you're back to square one again, every month.'

I asked her to start from the beginning. She met her husband, John, seven years ago, three weeks before her thirtieth birthday. Both big rugby fans, they happened to be in the same pub after watching a match at Twickenham in 2017.

'I knew on our third date that he was the one,' she smiled.

After a few months of getting to know each other they established that they both definitely wanted children, but John was in no rush.

'He takes things more slowly than me, and after two years I was like, could we start trying? But he wasn't quite ready yet. Because of my sister's fertility problems, I always said I didn't want to wait years.'

By this point, Aisling's older sister, Louise, and her husband, had been struggling with infertility for six years and Aisling worried she might have trouble conceiving too.

After three and a half years together, in December 2020, John agreed to start trying and Aisling had her coil removed.

'I was so excited, it was like an early Christmas present,' she said, before apologising at how 'stupid that sounds'. I told her I had felt the same when James and I started trying. There is a giddiness in finally letting nature do its thing – after over a decade of using contraception – and not knowing when or if it will work.

'But nothing happened. For over two years nothing happened.

I did the ovulation sticks, legs up in the air, different positions, all the things you read about; we tried it all.'

In February 2023 they were referred for IVF. Aisling was in the middle of her consultant training and had to inject herself every day while working intense shifts in the emergency unit.

'I was going into the toilet cubicle with my little sharps box and my medication, like in *Mean Girls* where she sits on the toilet seat with her lunch.'

At the egg retrieval, they collected eight eggs and the next day Aisling got a call to say that four had fertilised. But a few days later only two had continued to develop; one was frozen and the other was transferred into her uterus. Two weeks later she took a pregnancy test.

'John came out of the bathroom crying,' she said. 'I couldn't believe it. We'd never had a positive test, so we were over the moon.' Their wedding day was scheduled for a few months later.

'I was going to be pregnant on our wedding day . . . which is usually what people *don't* want,' she laughed. 'I thought, I'm gonna have to adjust my dress, but I didn't care.'

They went for a scan and heard the heartbeat, but were told that the embryo was measuring small and were recommended to have another scan in ten days.

'I couldn't wait ten days, so we paid for a private scan a few days later,' said Aisling. 'It was Easter Sunday and there was no heartbeat. They said unfortunately the baby had died. So obviously we were completely devastated, just beside ourselves.'

The hospital gave them three options: wait for the miscarriage to happen in its own time, take some medication or manage it surgically.

'It was my hen party the following weekend, so I was like whatever is the quickest option. I didn't want to be miscarrying on my hen weekend.'

My heart twisted with compassion. The timing of such events

is never ideal, but there's something extra painful about one such as this.

'The surgery went completely fine,' she continued, 'but I remember just as they were putting me to sleep, I started bawling my eyes out in the anaesthetic room. I thought about how empty I would be when I woke up.' Her voice wobbled, then broke. 'I'll never forget that image, you know. It makes me so sad to think about it again now.'

That summer Aisling and John got married and kept trying, hoping they might get pregnant on their honeymoon 'like everyone else seems to'. But when they didn't, they planned to have their frozen embryo transferred a few months later. In the meantime, to their surprise, they fell pregnant naturally. After nearly three years of trying, Aisling couldn't believe it.

They went for a six-week scan and were told that the embryo was measuring small again. Ten days later they had another scan, and then another.

'For about a month it dragged on. There was still a heartbeat, but it wasn't growing so I knew it wasn't going to end well. Then they mentioned it might be a molar pregnancy, so I had to have surgery again.'

Infertility is not black and white, I thought. It is not just about getting pregnant, but staying pregnant.

'I had the surgery on the Monday, and then on the Tuesday morning Sophie got her news.'

Sophie had been having migraines, facial numbness and anxiety for a few months. She visited her GP three times but each time was dismissed because they believed she was suffering from anxiety due to her stressful job. By the fourth appointment the GP finally agreed to refer her for an MRI scan. It revealed a large brain tumour – the size of a lime – at the base of her skull, wrapped around her pituitary gland. Doctors were surprised she hadn't been having seizures or lost her vision because it was pressing on her optic nerve. She would need a biopsy – a small bit of tumour pulled out through her nose – to determine if it was cancerous, and then a full craniotomy. Brain surgery.

Aisling helped Sophie translate the medical jargon and ensure that all the necessary scans and support were set in motion. For Sophie, it also brought her own fertility into question, but conversations about freezing her eggs were hijacked by conversations about just making sure she stayed alive.

'I don't think we ever really grieved that loss,' Aisling said of the miscarriage she suffered around Sophie's diagnosis. 'Things got put to the side for six months essentially. Everything with Sophie was so sad and so stressful, our stuff wasn't a priority any more.'

Four months later, after Sophie's surgery, Aisling and John had their frozen embryo transferred, but it didn't take.

'So we were back to square one. I took the day off work the next day because I was just so sad. I know it's only an embryo, but in your mind it's your baby. It was going to be our baby and our child.'

Two months later they got pregnant naturally again, but it also ended in miscarriage around seven weeks. Aisling had a hysteroscopy to look inside her womb and take a biopsy, which came back as normal. In the meantime John had another test for DNA fragmentation – which had initially come back as normal – but the re-test showed some abnormality.

'He got referred to a urologist and they said he's got varicocele.'

A varicocele is an enlarged vein in the scrotum, similar to a varicose vein in your leg. It can cause overheating of the testes, which can negatively impact sperm production and function. Approximately 10–15 per cent of men have a varicocele, but it's not routinely tested for during fertility investigations, even though it can be a cause of infertility and miscarriage. It is estimated that four in ten men who struggle to conceive their first child may have varicoceles, and a staggering eight out of ten men with secondary infertility. Treatment – an embolisation or surgery – is quick and safe.

'So what's next?' I asked.

'He had the procedure done last month, but the urologist said it'll take three months for his sperm to improve so now we're in this weird limbo place where I'm like, let's just try anyway but he's saying no, because we don't want to go through another miscarriage. So that's another few months we have to wait. I can see that yes, he's right, but it feels very unnatural to waste three months; in my mind that's a lot. I'm thirty-seven now.'

I felt for Aisling. Infertility involves delicate decision-making and careful coordination of work and a social life, all while time itself seems to be speeding up and conspiring against you.

'And obviously it's the cost,' she continued. 'The next round will be at least £15,000, which we're trying to save and then I need to plan time off work.'

I asked if she dealt with many pregnancies at work.

'I see people having miscarriages,' she replied, 'and I feel like I can show them a lot more empathy than other people. Very soon after my miscarriages I probably wasn't able to see them, but now I would actively choose to see those patients so that I can hopefully provide a better kind of comfort for them.'

Throughout our conversation we talked about how only other people who have been through infertility can truly understand it; how bonds can be made or broken when dealing with something that so many people come by easily, and perhaps take for granted. For Aisling, it has affected her friendships.

'One of my best friends, we've definitely grown distant now. Our relationship has changed. I'm going to her wedding soon and she'll be thirty-four weeks pregnant. I'm kind of dreading it because all our friends have got kids now so I'm gonna be the only one on that table without kids. I usually love weddings, but I'm more of a hermit now. I feel like a broken record, you know, I have nothing else really to say aside from no, we're still here, still trying, four years later. It's taken over my life, so I'm not really a fun person any more. It's hard not to feel resentful of everyone else.'

Some friends have stopped checking in with her after getting pregnant themselves – perhaps, Aisling thought, because they don't want to seem like they're rubbing it in – while others have made an effort to understand and messaged her sensitively.

'They know how difficult it's been and have sent me the most lovely messages saying I know this is going to be really difficult for you and I wanted to text you because I know that face-to-face can be really hard. But annoyingly, they've often texted at the start of a work day, during handover, which means trying really hard not to cry in front of everyone. But the nice messages show that they've thought about it and I always appreciate that.'

On a recent visit to Ireland, I visited Aisling's parents and stayed in her childhood bedroom; bright pink everything, just like mine used to be. Around the house were beautiful photos of the three sisters together. While Aisling and Orla now live in London, Louise has stayed in Ireland. I asked how Louise's fertility journey was going.

'She's forty-five now,' Aisling said. 'At one point, when she told me they needed to make a decision about whether they're gonna stop, I found it so sad.' Aisling's voice splintered as she tried to get her words out without crying. 'To think it might be the end of their journey. It's taken so long and just completely eaten away at them. They've had seven embryo transfers, so God knows how much money they've spent on it all.'

In terms of next steps, they have discussed surrogacy but Louise's husband is undecided.

'In Ireland fertility treatment is still very hush-hush and very gossipy,' Aisling said. 'There's an old Irish mentality, like, what will the neighbours think?'

I think about my parents keeping their secret from their own family, never mind the neighbours.

'Am I right in thinking the last few embryos were created from eggs donated by Orla?' I asked.

'Yes, that's right.'

While Louise was ready to move on to egg donation straight away, her husband took longer to digest the loss and grieve the fact they would no longer be using Louise's eggs. In the end, he agreed and was grateful that Louise had a younger sister who was willing to donate hers. Unfortunately, it didn't work. When I speak to Louise, later on, about her journey, she reiterates that they will be forever grateful to Orla for giving them more chances.

After more than a decade of trying, Louise and her husband have never had a positive pregnancy test. I told Aisling that one of the reasons I wanted to talk to her was because we only ever hear of the happy ending stories – tending to be bombarded with them by well-meaning friends – and I wanted to mention the other stories; the ones that don't end with a baby and the ones that aren't finished yet.

'A friend I went to medical school with had been trying for five years, and we both got pregnant at the same time,' Aisling said. 'Me from the IVF, and she was about to start IVF and got pregnant naturally. She was one of those really annoying stories.' We both laugh.

'They are so annoying,' I said, 'and yet I really hope that will be us one day.' Aisling nodded.

Aisling and John tried for six more months before starting another expensive round of IVF. This time they paid extra for Preimplantation Genetic Testing for Aneuploidy (PGT-A), a genetic test to screen embryos for chromosomal abnormalities. The transferred embryo was confirmed to be euploid (normal) but a few weeks later Aisling miscarried again.

In the years since their daughter was born, Tim and Gina have tried for a sibling and also endured multiple miscarriages. A year after her brain surgery, Sophie's treatment has not concluded; her life is still on hold. The tumour was not cancerous, but since the bulk of it was removed, it has continued to grow and cause problems. Louise, Aisling and I are still waiting for our time. We are all living in a state of limbo.

Christmas

Definition

1. A Christian holy day to honour the birth of Jesus
2. December 25th

In my family, I'm the one who loves Christmas the most. Growing up, every year around the end of November, I begged Mum to let me put up the Christmas tree. One of my favourite tasks was assembling the Nativity scene by the window down the hallway. It was an annual routine that I savoured. First I would clean the wooden ledge with a cloth and polish, leaving a scent of delicious waxy leather. Next I would lift the Nativity set out of the storage box, pulling out clumps of straw from the wicker basket and flatten it down with my hands. It smelled sweet and musty. I would gently lay out the colourful ceramic figurines that had been waiting patiently all year for their time to shine. Baby Jesus in his cot was always the first to be nestled in the straw, with everyone else positioned around him: Mary, Joseph, the stable boy, the cow, the sheep and the goat. There wasn't enough room for the three wise men on the straw, so I lined them up just outside, looking in. That's how religion has always felt for me. I'm enchanted by the stories, but always on the outside, looking in.

Because I enjoy Christmas so much, Mum always asked me to write the Christmas cards to our friends and relatives. I happily obliged, relishing the responsibility of choosing each card from a miscellaneous box she had amassed over the years. Every year, inside the box was the same crumpled piece of lined paper: a handwritten list of names and addresses. Written next to each name was either 'and family' or not, depending on whether they had children. Against one couple, Anne and Chris, in capital, red, underlined letters, were the words: NOT AND FAMILY.

Despite the clear instructions, Mum always used to check that I hadn't written 'and family' in their Christmas card.

'No, don't worry,' I would say.

'You know the story, don't you?'

'Yes, I know.'

When my parents were expecting Tim, their neighbour was in the process of adopting a child, and their social worker, Anne, mentioned that she and her husband were having trouble getting pregnant. The neighbour told Anne that Sandra, next door, had gotten pregnant via IVF and when she introduced them, Sandra and Anne became friends. The following year Anne also got pregnant via IVF and gave birth to a baby girl called Donna.

Anne and Chris got on well with their milkman and he would pop over for a cup of tea in between his rounds each morning. When he left, little toddler Donna would run outside and wave him off excitedly, which everyone found adorable. One day, when Donna was eighteen months old, she ran out to wave goodbye, but that morning, as he was reversing the float, the milkman didn't see her.

My parents went to Donna's funeral and have never forgotten the image of her tiny coffin. It is one of the saddest stories I have ever heard.

In the years that followed, Anne and Chris tried IVF again several times, staying with John and Sandra each time as they lived closer to the clinic. Sandra delayed her next round of IVF because the thought of getting pregnant again before Anne was unthinkable. But each round failed. Years later Anne did get pregnant again, naturally, but it was ectopic. They never had any more children and she died a few years ago.

One of the injustices of infertility is the added anxiety for some that after all the heartache and effort and money and time it has taken to get pregnant that one day it might all be taken away. When my friend Alice gave birth to her IVF baby, the birth was traumatic and life-threatening. Her son was premature, small and fragile, and Alice felt overwhelmed with the responsibility of keeping him alive. She experienced such excruciating postpartum depression that she questioned if she was even meant to be a mother, and whether she should go on living.

'Thoughts were flashing constantly through my mind,' she wrote in a beautiful Substack post. 'This is why we couldn't conceive without fertility treatment. This is why we nearly both died when he was born. This is where my luck runs out. The universe had tried damn hard to tell me but stupid me ignored the signs. Now I had to face up to the hard truth.'

'But,' she continued, 'that wasn't the truth.'

In heightened states of upheaval, our minds can play tricks on us, convincing us of terrible things that bear little grounding in reality. Since I discovered my origins and tried to make sense of the secrecy surrounding it, I have grappled with what we mean by 'the truth' and what we should do with it.

Then you will know the truth and the truth will set you free – John, 8:32.

But what if the truth does not set us free? What if the truth creates more trauma?

I do not know if the fertility clinic encouraged my parents to lie to us, or whether doing that was so commonplace that it was barely a conversation worth having. Doctors were there to solve medical problems, not advise parents on the individual ethics of keeping secrets. Unless there was an obvious need to tell the children, why bother? Children believe what they are told and adults are just doing their best to help their kids fit in and feel normal. How different, really, is the secret of a sperm donor to the lies, the untruths, we tell our children about the tooth fairy or Santa Claus?

I woke up on Christmas morning 2022 and started crying. It was like a geyser had been building pressure inside my head and suddenly erupted. A few months earlier I had made the decision to tell my siblings the truth and the perfect opportunity had presented itself. We had all arranged to meet at Tim and Gina's house a few days after Christmas. Our parents wouldn't be there, which was important; I didn't want anyone to have to worry about Mum and Dad's feelings on top of their own.

'What's the matter?' James asked, as I sat up in bed, tears streaming silently down my face.

'I'm so worried about telling them,' I replied. 'It just feels more real now.' James hugged me and we agreed to take the morning slowly, at my pace. We were at his parents' house – hundreds of miles away from mine – and it was the first time I'd ever spent Christmas Day away from my family. I was missing them.

As we headed downstairs, James's mum returned from church.

'How was it?' James asked.

She explained to me that it was something she did every year, mostly out of nostalgia. Even though she was not religious herself, her father had been a vicar.

'It was lovely,' she said. 'I have lots of happy memories as a little girl going to church on Christmas Day. But it's sad too.' Her eyes were red and wet. 'Because it makes me miss him.' She wiped away tears.

We enjoyed a beautiful Christmas dinner and, embraced by James's family and their traditions, I was distracted from my own worries for a while. But when we went for a walk along the seafront we saw a dead seal lying on the beach and it felt like a bad omen.

Twelve days earlier, in a last-minute panic, I had emailed the Donor Conception Network, a charity dedicated to supporting donor conception families, asking for advice. I received a kind and empathetic reply from Nina, the director, and a link to a booklet aimed at parents deciding to tell their adult children. There was no booklet for siblings telling siblings.

The booklet was enlightening and made me feel emotional unexpectedly. It explained that parents needed to face their own difficult feelings first, in order to be able to listen to their children's feelings and not focus on their own. But back when I was conceived, it seemed that sweeping things under the carpet was the more typical approach. 'Without the opportunity to discuss feelings and mourn the loss of their fertility,' the booklet read, 'many men were left feeling that their infertility was a personal failure and something to be ashamed of. Some men may still feel this way.'

My parents needed to grieve the children they did not have, and I'm not sure they ever did. We had been so wanted, but there was loss there too. These hard conversations had to be had; I needed to break the generational cycle of silence.

Two days later it was finally D-Day, as I called it: Donor Day. After a better night's sleep, I felt calm and resolute. We said our goodbyes to James's family and drove seventy miles north to Tim and Gina's house.

When we arrived, everyone else and their partners were already there. As we hugged I felt relieved that logistically the plan had come to fruition, but I was also simmering with dread. Tim and Gina had booked a meal at a local pub, and we had some time to catch up before heading out. We settled into the living room where my two-year-old niece, Ava, was playing with her toys on the floor. James and I sat near the fireplace. I looked around and thought about how this room was about to become forever engulfed in this memory. James held my hand and nodded. After 1,401 days of keeping the secret, it was time.

'Before we go out,' I said. 'I've got something I want to talk to everyone about.'

'Oh god,' Joe mumbled. The room fell silent. Everyone looked at me.

'There's no good time or place to do it, but we're all here together.' I felt dizzy. The dark blue walls felt like a giant whirlpool, spinning me around, with no way out.

'Sorry to sound dramatic. Nobody's dying, everything's okay.' I paused. I had no script, I had decided to just let the truth tumble out however it wanted to.

'I need to get it off my mind, because it's been difficult.' My mouth was moving, but my mind was willing it shut.

'This might be a surprise to everyone, but basically, a few years ago, you all know that I signed up to that DNA kit thing?' They nodded. 'And that was all fine, and then a few years later, something surprising came up. And I spoke to Mum and Dad about it and then we sort of . . . didn't talk about it for a long time, but it's got to the point now where I just feel like we should all talk about it . . .' I tried to keep breathing. '. . . In a nice, loving space, while we're all together, without them here. And nothing has to change.'

Everyone looked terrified. I just needed to get the words out.

'When Mum and Dad needed IVF, Mum had endometriosis, as you all know, which meant that she couldn't conceive naturally. But they also found that Dad's sperm wasn't viable. So, to create us, they used a sperm donor.'

I paused and waited for the outpouring. The screams, the gasps, the tears. But none came. Just a few murmurs of surprise. Everyone was still looking at me and listening intently.

'And I know that's very unexpected to hear,' I continued, 'and obviously it doesn't change anything. Dad is Dad. And Mum and Dad really, really, really wanted us.' There were whispers of agreement. 'And we've had such a great, happy family and childhood.'

'Yeah,' Ruth said.

'We have,' Tim chimed in.

'And they decided not to tell us, and for years that was fine. But ironically I did a DNA test to check where Dad's birth parents were from, because obviously none of us know. And then this came out.' No one said anything. There was still such an absence of emotion, I didn't know whether to keep talking or not.

'And when I found out, they wanted to tell everyone, but it was Easter weekend and I'd planned an egg hunt and I just couldn't handle it at the time. I didn't know whether we would have the conversation again, or whether they would tell you. But they haven't.'

'Do they know that you're telling everyone now?' Gina asked.

'No,' I said. 'And the reason is because I think it was quite hard for them. Dad got upset and afterwards he came and spoke to me and just said, nothing's changed, has it? And I said, no, you're always our dad . . . if anything it makes me realise that you wanted us more.'

'Thanks for telling us Bex, you've been sitting on that,' Ruth said eventually. 'It must have been such a burden.'

'That's a lot for one person to carry,' added Gina. 'It's a massive thing.'

'So did they use the same sperm donor for everyone?' Tim asked and my heart dropped. I knew this would be one of the first questions.

'Okay, so I've obviously only done the DNA test myself, but as far as I'm aware, I think us three have the same donor and Tim has a different donor.'

Tim looked down. I hated the thought of othering him, as if us being triplets wasn't enough.

I told them about Lucy getting in contact and meeting Libby too. I told them about the donor joining the DNA website a year later. They asked questions and I did my best to answer them. Nobody seemed traumatised. I felt relieved, and uneasy. Perhaps it would be a slow burn and the emotion would ignite later. I couldn't relax yet.

'Well, we've got the most complicated family tree ever,' Tim said and everyone laughed.

'Shall we all have a drink?' said James, and everyone laughed again.

'Why don't we go and pour ourselves a big glass of wine and we'll cheers to an amazing family,' Gina said. 'And can I just say, I feel blessed to be a part of this family, and I feel blessed that I get to make it bigger and, one day maybe there'll be some more cousins to join in, but your dad is the top of a family tree and it's an incredible family to be a part of. It's a family that couldn't be more wanted.'

'Thank you, Gina,' I said. Her words were a great comfort.

'Oh, I've got something for everyone,' I suddenly remembered. 'I made coasters with photos of the four of us and you can each choose one to keep.'

Tim, Ruth and Joe gathered around and looked at the coasters on the table. Four different photos of us as children, together. One in front of Stonehenge, one at Land's End, one in our kitchen, and another re-enacting *The Lion King* on 'pride rock' at Cheddar Gorge.

'This is just to remind us that we're all in it together, okay?' I said as we hugged. 'We always have each other.'

'I think we should tell Mum and Dad that we know,' Tim said and Ruth and Joe nodded. 'It's best not to have any more secrets.'

Concrete

Definition

1. Existing in physical form
2. A building material
3. Clear and certain

We agreed to tell Mum and Dad the next time we gathered together as a family, a few months later for Easter weekend. But first we were put to work. Mum and Dad had asked all of us, plus partners, to help them lay the foundations for the 'garden room': an extension of the house they'd been planning for fifteen years. So slow was the progress of this conservatory that it had taken on mythical status; we joked it would never get done.

It was a crisp morning so we wrapped up in fleeces, woolly hats and wellies. Around 9 a.m. a man in an orange high-vis jacket turned up, with a colossal concrete mixing truck rumbling behind him. Dad had constructed a large wooden holding pen, lined with polythene, on the driveway because the extension was at the rear of the house, with no accessible route for a vehicle. The plan was to wheelbarrow the wet concrete around in loads. The high-vis man pressed a button and the bowels of the truck opened. A slurry of grey slush began to drop from the tunnel attached to the rotating belly, plopping slowly into the pen like giant diarrhoea.

Concrete is made of cement, water and aggregates – like gravel, sand or rock – and it is not to be messed with. Concrete is poured and shaped when wet and in a matter of hours it sets and hardens. Once the cement binds with water, it begins a chain reaction that cannot be reversed. One thing forever becomes another. There is no going back.

I knew it would be the same if we told Dad. The thought of bringing it all up again made me feel sick, but one secret had multiplied, and now there was a labyrinth of half-lies. We just needed to jump this last hurdle.

All ten of us got to work, shovelling and wheeling and pouring. Ava wore a penguin bobble hat and was propped up on a big bag of sand. She wanted to help too. Using a small yellow plastic shovel, she carefully moved sand from one side of the bag to the other. When we needed a breather between wheelbarrows, we took it in turns to encourage her with her very important shovelling.

Dad stationed himself in the garden room, telling us where to pour our wheelbarrows and then, on his hands and knees, started spreading out the concrete evenly using a wooden float. Ruth squatted next to him, keeping it level with a long piece of timber.

Throughout the morning I checked in with everyone individually, making sure they were still happy with the plan to tell Mum and Dad. Yes, they said. I felt a rush of anticipation that finally everything would be out in the open.

I was impressed that Mum, at seventy-one years old, was just as quick and capable of doing the tough physical work as the rest of us. Initially, shovelling the concrete was easy – like spooning peanut butter from a new tub – but after two hours of ferrying back and forth, it resembled the bottom of the jar: crunchy, stiff and bone-achingly heavy to scoop. But concrete waits for no one; we had to keep going until it was done.

If blood is thicker than water, concrete is thicker than both. It is the second most used substance in the world, after water. For thousands of years we have relied on it for shelter and safety, for transport and flooring. The Greeks, Romans and Mayans used it to build temples, amphitheatres and aqueducts. It is ubiquitous, solid and enduring. It holds time at bay. Concrete protects us, but it also entombs us and we have buttressed ourselves against nature with it, marking our territory on this planet with giant grey slabs. It has turned our world from green to grey. Concrete cannot soak up storms and floods like soil can. It cannot feed and sustain life; it disrupts the ecosystem. We put up these walls, only to find we can't see through them.

Around 2 p.m. we stopped for lunch and gathered to admire the new floor, proud of what we had achieved. The concrete was a smooth and luminous grey, reflecting the last of the light, latticed through the window panes. I thought our duties were done, but Dad said he wanted a few of us to help resurface the paths around the house with the leftover concrete and sand. Breaking our news would have to wait.

By the time we'd finished, it was dark and dinner was almost ready. As a family, we have barbecues all year round, keeping warm by the fire pit as we wait for the grill to heat up behind us. I grabbed a beer and sat down with everyone.

'How are your knees, Dad?' Ruth asked. He had been kneeling down all day, not easy for a seventy-two-year-old. I assumed that's what she was talking about.

'They're sore,' he replied. 'It was silly of me really, I should've known better.'

'Why, what happened?' I asked.

'Dad's knees got burnt,' Joe replied. 'Chemical burns from the concrete. It's quite bad.'

The wet concrete had soaked through his trousers and burned his skin as it dried. Mum showed me a photo she'd taken on her phone, his knees a screaming raw bullseye of redness. I felt a twinge of pain and deep empathy – how I imagine a parent feels when their child gets injured on the playground – a sudden awareness of the fragility of someone you love. It turned out that my dad – so strong, skilful and impressive in his work – had delicate skin on his knees just like the rest of us.

I could see that Dad was mad with himself. He'd been in the building trade for fifty years; he knew he should have worn knee pads. Everything had gone perfectly aside from this one mishap, one from which he alone would have to bear the slow agony of healing.

With Dad's blistered knees, all of our aching bodies and the growing lateness of the evening, it was clearly not the right time to talk about things. The foundations had been laid; we would go to bed and broach it the next day.

We had a slow Sunday morning; resurfacing from our rooms and pulled towards the smell of bacon and eggs cooking in the kitchen. As it was Easter weekend, we played our annual games and egg hunt, but as the day drew on, I worried we were never going to get round to talking to Dad.

Finally, after a very long Easter quiz, it seemed like our opportunity had arrived. Dad was in the living room watching a documentary about an unsolved murder. I darted around the house, asking everyone's partners if they would mind heading to the kitchen and waiting there while we talked to our parents in the living room in private. They nodded, said they'd keep themselves entertained and to take as long as we needed. I herded my siblings into the living room.

Dad was sitting in the same chair as last time. I perched behind him, on the same sofa as before; it wasn't intentional, it just happened that way. As everyone else sat down, I tried to ignore the feeling of wanting to run away.

'John, can you just turn off the television for a minute,' Mum said. 'They want to talk to you.'

Dad reached for the remote and pressed mute. A rigid silence descended. I looked around to see everyone else staring at the floor. I realised it would have to be me who spoke first. Me, again, who plunged the knife. For a few moments I was furious, indignant. I felt stupid for not thinking this far ahead and asking someone else to speak first. I was so tired of trying to word bad news well. I wanted it to be a joint statement, a unanimous decision, a problem shared, but it felt like I was alone again.

'Dad, we have something we want to talk to you about,' I said.

He grunted and half looked over at us, realising that the door was closed.

'A few months ago I told everyone . . . about how we were conceived.'

'What?' Dad jolted up in his seat.

'I didn't think it was right to keep it a secret from everyone.'

'Right,' Dad replied softly, then turned to Mum. 'Did you know?'

'I didn't know she was going to tell them,' Mum replied. 'I had no idea.'

It felt accusatory, like he was looking for someone to blame, but I'm not sure what it was. I realised that for Dad this must have felt a bit like an ambush. He wanted to check his own wife had not kept him in the dark. No, it was just me: the rogue daughter. All because I selfishly couldn't keep a secret any longer.

Dad closed his eyes and shielded his face with his hand, like before. He had just been trying to relax after a busy weekend and here we were, inflicting this on him. I had naively assumed that one of us knowing was not so different from all of us knowing, but I was wrong. He didn't want all of us to know. Sharing the secret with my siblings was not a relief for him, as I'd hoped, but another injury. Three more stabs to his side, just as the last one had healed into a scar.

I looked around and asked my siblings for support with my eyes. *Come on, someone else say something.*

'It's okay, Dad,' said Tim, finally. 'It doesn't change anything. We still love you. It's better for us to know.'

Ruth and I went over to hug him, but he didn't move. I felt helpless. I knew I had done the right thing – or at least not the wrong thing – but I had expected it to feel better. The weight was shared now, I thought, though the guilt was not.

We had waited all weekend to say something, and I understood why, but it meant we all departed soon after the conversation, back to our own homes and lives. I got the sense that Dad wanted to be left alone with his emotions for a while, though I worried he would feel like we were deserting him. When we said our goodbyes, I hugged him, but he barely hugged me back. I told him I loved him, but he didn't say it back. James and I got in the car and drove back up north. I ached with sadness.

The next morning I went litter picking at my local park with a volunteer group. It felt good to be in nature and get some headspace, but as I pincered crisp packets and dirty tissues from the ground, my head was spinning with undigested emotions. Everyone knew now, I kept telling myself, and that was all I wanted. Still, I felt groggy and hungover. I didn't regret what I'd done, I just wished I hadn't had to do it. It was like putting a half-dead animal out of its misery; necessary but cruel.

As I picked up individual cigarette butts with my picker, I looked into the lake ahead. A handful of swans were bobbing a few metres away, too early for cygnets.

I pulled my phone out of my pocket and texted Mum.

Is dad okay?

**He's very quiet. Not mentioned anything.
I'll wait until he feels like talking himself.**

Yeah good idea. I feel so bad about it all. I don't ever want to make him upset.

> It goes back further than you finding out.
> So don't feel bad.
>
> It's something that was always going to need addressing.
>
> It'll be fine when he's absorbed it all and sees nothing's changed.
>
> Better for everyone now it's out in the open. You're all amazing and have taken it so well.

I knew Dad had lived through some difficult family dynamics growing up. When he was a child, his dad left his mum for another woman. At the time his parents had been fostering a little girl called Lorraine and were in the process of adopting her. John loved having a sibling but when his dad left, she was abruptly taken away and John never saw her again.

After his parents' separation, John stopped seeing his dad so often and by the time he was eighteen it had been a few years. He knew where his dad had moved to and one day knocked on the door unannounced. But John wasn't invited in. His dad had a new family and John had to accept that he wouldn't be a part of it. He never got to introduce him to his fiancé, Sandra. A month before their wedding, his dad died from a heart attack.

I felt some relief at knowing there was more to his reaction than just our revelation, but I was still heartbroken at the thought of him brewing and brooding on his own.

Later that day, I drove 150 miles south to a small village on the Welsh border. I had booked the week off work to attend a tutored writing retreat. It was the first time I would tell my story out loud to strangers.

Swimmers

Definition

1. People that swim
2. Swimming costume
3. Sperm

Fingers together like a paddle, my shoulders rotate for every slice of hand before sculling through the silk. My head is still like a rudder – eyes on the ceiling – as I glide along an invisible twine, avoiding the lane rope, sharper than it looks. As the end approaches, I tuck my body into itself, like a foetus, and push my feet against the tiles. Each turn a springboard, propelling me forward, as I kick rhythmically into a new length.

As children, we spent a lot of time in water, swimming competitively from the age of nine. My favourite stroke was, and still is, backstroke. Some people don't like it because you can't see where you're going, but from a young age I built up a kind of braveness. I liked having to trust myself; the gamble each length that I hadn't misjudged my speed when counting strokes from the flags: five at a casual pace, three when sprinting. Time it wrong and you smash your head into the wall.

The Coxon triplets were always late for everything, but being late for swimming was the worst. On Thursday evenings, there were five words I dreaded hearing Mum say.

'Get changed in the car.'

We would groan and whine in protest.

'You'll be late otherwise,' she said. 'It means you can jump straight into the pool.'

We did as we were told, grabbing our swimsuits from our bags and trying to manoeuvre our bodies into them – all while in the back of a moving car, trying not to expose ourselves to innocent bystanders on the street.

The leisure centre car park was often busy, with cars backed up around the entrance, so Mum would accelerate to the far end, swerve and brake.

'You'll have to get out here,' she'd shout. Reluctantly we opened the doors and stepped out, barefoot, on to the sharp gravelly ground. Wearing just our swimming costumes – goggles and hats in hand – we ran as fast as we could across the tarmac, bracing the cold and ignoring the stares of bewildered onlookers. We rushed through the doors, past reception, straight on to poolside and launched ourselves into the water, as if we'd always been there.

Almost every weekend was a club, county or national competition and each time we'd bring home a cluster of trophies and medals, lining them up on the kitchen table in height order. Gold, silver, bronze. We all happened to be best at different strokes, to our parents' relief, because it meant we rarely competed directly against each other.

We competed in other sports too. Tennis, netball, cheerleading, football. There was always a training session or match to ferry us to and from. One year Ruth and I both made it to the final of our school's annual tennis competition. It was like Serena versus Venus: Ruth versus Rebecca. I won, but I'll never forget the car ride home, as we sat in silence, Ruth and I both staring out the window, me grinning and clutching my trophy, Ruth quietly sobbing. Our parents not knowing what to do.

For a sperm to reach an egg, it has to swim the equivalent of thirty miles in relation to its size, more than a marathon.

They use their flagella – whip-like tails – to swim in a corkscrew motion. Though it's more like digging and nudging and squirming than swimming, and more like thick jelly than the water in a swimming pool. Most get lost and the ones that don't have only a 50 per cent chance of choosing the fallopian tube that contains the egg.

Within eight seconds of the semen entering the vagina, the pH level of the upper vagina is raised to match the sperm, making it a less hostile environment for them. Around the same time the semen becomes a gel, or coagulum. Around thirty to sixty minutes later, the gel degrades, and the sperm can start to swim again.

Some sperm are good at swimming forward, but most are not. The majority cannot swim in a straight line, while others struggle to move at all. This swimming ability is called motility. The vast majority of sperm are also defective in shape or size. Some have heads that are too small, large or misshapen, while others have two heads. Some have tails that are crooked or short or broken; others have two tails and a few have no tails at all. This variation in appearance is called morphology. For most men, at least 90 per cent of their sperm will have abnormal morphology.

Sperm volume is the number of millilitres of ejaculate produced, while sperm count refers to the concentration of sperm. A low sperm count contains less than fifteen million sperm per millilitre. Some people have no sperm in their semen at all, which is known as azoospermia. As men grow older, all these measures of sperm competency decrease. Men over forty are 30 per cent less likely to conceive than men under thirty. The more I learn about the intricacies of natural conception, the more unlikely it seems.

As James and I started trying to conceive, each month around ovulation I noticed my body getting inflamed and sore. It felt like my immune system was kicking into action every time we had sex, destroying any trespassers. I pictured a 1980s arcade game of Space Invaders or Pac-Man. The sperm were trying to navigate the maze of my pelvis, but the gang of ghosts – my white blood cells – were always wiping them out. Anxious that we weren't getting pregnant and my endometriosis was getting worse, I went to my GP who conducted a blood test. It revealed, as expected, that my AMH level – an indicator of how many eggs you have left – had decreased. I was only thirty-one, but disheartened to learn that I had the ovarian reserve of a forty-year-old. The GP referred me to the local fertility clinic but warned that the waiting time was at least seven months long, and that was just to start investigative tests, not treatment.

I searched online and discovered that if you paid for the tests privately, the process moved quicker and you still qualified for a free round of IVF treatment on the NHS, should you need it. I spoke to James and he agreed to split the costs fifty-fifty.

Initial testing revealed that the issue most likely lay with me, so that summer I put my researching skills to good use. I studied articles and science journals to learn how to improve my egg quality. I started using ovulation sticks and buying supplements. We ramped up sex around ovulation, ate even more healthily and I stopped drinking alcohol completely. I read books and listened to podcasts about fertility and started a course of acupuncture. It all added up financially, but I knew it would be worth it if it increased our chances.

I paid for a HyCoSy (Hysterosalpingo Contrast Sonography) test to check if my fallopian tubes were blocked. My tubes were clear, but according to the consultant this did not mean they were necessarily functioning properly. She said it was likely that my endometriosis was impacting our ability to conceive and referred us for IVF. Our local clinic happened to be part of the group that Simon Fishel founded, which felt fitting.

'Don't you think we should try naturally for a bit longer?' James asked me one evening, a few months later.

'They've already referred us for IVF. It would be crazy to turn it down now,' I snapped at him. 'I don't want to mess them about.' I was incensed that he was suggesting this after years of delaying us already.

'But we haven't been trying for that long,' he said.

'My endo is getting worse, I can't live with it. Plus there's only a 35 per cent chance of IVF working anyway,' I sighed. 'I'm ready and I just don't mentally feel like I can wait any longer.'

'But you don't *know* that you can't get pregnant naturally.'

He was right. I had no idea; no one did. All I had was a bleak diagnosis from two doctors, a genetic predisposition and a year's worth of periods to show for it. But everyone knew about improbable success stories. Miracle babies, conceived from couples told there was no hope.

To me, it felt like James wanted a 'natural' baby and believed that IVF was trying too hard. As a child of IVF, I was annoyed at his naivety. We were lucky to be offered IVF – how could we not take it? In any case, it was *my* body that was going to bear the physical brunt of it – alongside the weekly torment of my endometriosis symptoms – surely it was for *me* to decide when we did it? The conversation got heated and I shut it down.

For me, the timing was ideal. I was due to finish my TV work in October and start a Master's degree in creative writing. I would have more time and mental space to nurture a pregnancy, or keep trying IVF if needed. I was so pleased that things were finally moving forward.

Over the following weeks, we read pamphlets and watched educational videos sent to us by the clinic. We did blood tests and signed reams of paperwork that included our preferences about what would happen to our embryos if one of us died or became mentally incapacitated.

The day after Ruth's wedding, I started the IVF medication. For two weeks I took a pill three times a day that was designed to shut down my hormones. It made me feel on the edge of tears constantly, which was difficult while working in a job already humming with emotion.

James and I were both employed on a documentary series that followed hospital staff and patients at a busy accident and emergency department, filmed in my hometown of Nottingham. Part of my role was to interview patients and uncover interesting backstories to make the episodes feel as powerful and heartwarming as possible. I figured it was okay if I cried during the interviews with patients and their loved ones, but it was the other times that felt embarrassing. One lunchtime I was waiting to order at a café when a lady pushed in front of me. I said something, but she barked back at me. The server just shrugged and took her order first. I walked out of the café and burst into tears. A few days later I heard that a friend's kitten had died and I couldn't stop crying. I felt so fragile. It was unnerving to have such little control over my emotions.

The following week a friend got engaged – a gorgeous proposal from her boyfriend involving hundreds of yellow roses – and it sent me into a spiral of sadness for a few days. I was delighted for her, but it was another reminder of what I felt so far away from. I was sad that my life had not followed the trajectory of getting married and then having a baby, as I'd always imagined. As the possibility of becoming pregnant drew closer, I was grieving the traditional order of things, but when I hinted about this to James, I could tell he felt pressured and uncomfortable.

'Just give it time,' he would say, or, 'Why don't you propose to me?', which made me feel conflicted. Why was it always up to the man to propose? And yet, like most women, I had always envisioned a romantic, surprise proposal from my future husband. Along with committing to a relationship, moving in with each other, booking holidays and forging ahead with the tests and IVF, it felt like another thing that James wanted *me* to organise, but I was exhausted by having to always take the lead. Sometimes it felt like I was just towing him along behind me.

I had hoped he might propose on our three-week trip to New Zealand five months earlier. The thought had crossed my mind every time our campervan pulled up to a beautiful lake straddled by snow-capped mountains, illuminated by the sun. But he didn't, and with no other trips planned I didn't have high hopes for a proposal in the near future. I felt paranoid that certain people were looking down on me for this; for not being married or engaged before trying for a baby, which seemed unfair. It wasn't that I didn't want those things.

Two weeks later, it was a relief to begin the IVF injections, which had fewer side effects than the tablets. Every time I plunged the needle into my pinched belly fat, James stayed nearby in case I felt faint and brought me ice cubes to help with the itchy pelts of skin that sprouted from the injection site. Each stab was a step closer towards our much-wanted child.

I kept asking James how he was feeling about it all.

'I'm nervous,' he said, 'but excited.'

'Me too,' I replied.

Two years earlier, James had bought me a young apple tree as a Christmas present. While taking my IVF medication, we noticed that the tree was fruiting for the first time. I went outside and gently tugged a round apple from a branch, holding it in the palm of my hand for a moment, feeling proud. Our first, delicious apple. I brought the apple in and asked James if he wanted to try it first. He said yes and I took a video on my phone, hoping it would be a funny memory to look back on, hopefully coinciding with the conception of our child. Something that was ours; that we had patiently grown together.

He took a bite and winced. His eyes squinted and he comically exaggerated his chewing.

'How's the apple?' I asked, laughing.

'It's super sour,' he replied, then gagged.

That's when the video cuts out.

Frozen

Definition

1. Incapable of being changed or undone
2. Stored at a very low temperature
3. Feeling unable to move, usually because of fear

On Friday 8 September 2023, James bought me flowers. It was a beautifully arranged bouquet from a local florist, wrapped in brown paper. Pink and yellow dahlias, purple carnations and eucalyptus. He took a photo of me holding them outside our house. I'm wearing mint-coloured linen trousers and a striped top. My blonde hair is damp from the shower and I'm smiling. I look happy.

I had been injecting my belly for six days and was feeling surprisingly good. That evening my friend Lucy and her new boyfriend, Paul, were coming up to visit us for the weekend. The IVF process was drawing to an end and I was looking forward to the next stages, especially the embryo transfer. I had done everything else two and a half years earlier when I donated my eggs, and was excited that this time, finally, it was going to be my turn to have an embryo in my womb.

I realised that if everything went well, the dates would fall perfectly for telling our families over Christmas, three months later. Only my mum and a couple of friends knew we were doing the IVF. We thought it would be fun to keep it a total surprise for James's parents, who would become grandparents for the first time. I imagined their faces when we revealed the news, the celebrations that would ensue, a Christmas of even more joy. I had seen the way James's family doted on his young cousin and knew they'd be so excited about a grandchild of their own. Alongside the stresses of working full-time, fitting in fertility clinic appointments and starting a Master's degree, I was quietly fizzing with anticipation about our future. I worked out the date: it would be early June, a summer baby.

As the evening approached, I noticed that James was behaving oddly. We were both working from home but he kept leaving the house to get some fresh air, disappearing for thirty or forty minutes at a time. He seemed unsettled and restless. I asked if there was anything wrong, but he kept saying he was fine. I carried on with my work and around 5.30 p.m., as I was wrapping up for the day, he said he needed to talk. He was sitting on the sofa behind me, so I turned around from my desk.

'What is it?'

'I'm really sorry, Bex.' He looked terrified. 'But I don't think I can go through with it.'

'With what?' I said. 'The IVF?'

'Yes.'

But it was too late to change our minds, maybe he didn't realise that. I was two-thirds of the way through a schedule of drugs. We had signed legal forms, the hospital had a plan in place; it was all happening next week.

'It's a big decision,' I said calmly. 'I've been feeling nervous too.'

'I know, but I can't go through with it,' he repeated.

My gut clenched. He was getting cold feet, natural for anyone confronted with imminent parenthood. He just needed a sounding board; to lay out his worries and for me to listen and reassure him.

'Okay, what is it that's making you think that?'

'I've been feeling so anxious all day. I've never felt like this before. I can't just ignore how I'm feeling.'

I mustered all the empathy I could find. 'That's normal, James. It's a life-changing thing to do.'

'It's too soon for a baby,' he said. 'June is too soon.'

'But, James, this is our only free round of IVF. We can't delay it now, I've already used most of the medication. It cost thousands of pounds.'

'I know, I'm really sorry.'

My mind scrambled to figure out how this crisis could be resolved. It came out of the blue, it could disappear quickly too.

'But we've been trying for months and months,' I said. 'I've been off the pill for years. I don't understand how this is any different.'

'I know,' he said, looking at the floor. 'I'm sorry.'

A quiet rage sizzled inside me again, the one telling me he thought IVF was unnecessary or unnatural; forcing it.

'I've been on the phone to people, talking it through,' he continued.

I wheezed with horror. 'What about the surprise?' I couldn't understand why he was ruining the surprise for his family.

'Wait—' my throat tightened. 'Just to be clear. Do you not want children now, or ever, or just not with me?'

'I don't know,' he said.

I stared at him, the man I had loved for more than three years. His young, handsome face looked older and more tired. He was clearly very stressed. Had he just gone along with the IVF to appease me? Did he actually want to do it? I suddenly felt like I didn't know him at all, and also, painfully, like I should have seen this coming.

James was a self-confessed people pleaser; he often agreed to things on the spot or over-promised in order to avoid conflict. I saw it in his work life, his friendships and our relationship, and it had been a character point of contention for us from the beginning. But this was too important. Why, after years of telling me he wasn't ready to start trying, would he agree only to change his mind again?

Then I realised, this might not just be about children.

'Do you still want to be with me?' I asked.

'Yes, I want to be with you, but I'm feeling so scared about it all.' He looked like he might cry. 'I've barely done any work today, I've felt so physically anxious in my body. I feel sick. I can't ignore it, Bex.'

I felt for him, his anguish was palpable. But my sense of injustice overrode it. How could one day of anxiety about having a child outweigh the years of anxiety I'd had about *never* being able to have one? Every day that my body ached from endometriosis, the sleepless nights, worrying that my chances were subsiding every passing year. The ball was always in his court, and still, he was telling me, he wasn't ready.

'Is it just today you've been feeling like this?'

'No. It's been a few weeks. Maybe a few months,' he replied.

'Oh my god. Why didn't you say something?'

'I'm sorry. I didn't have the courage to tell you. I was worried about how you would react.'

Every part of me panicked. 'But, I don't understand. Telling me now is *so* much worse. The egg collection is in a few days, how could you have not said anything?'

'I'm so sorry.'

My tear ducts burst open and the next hour brought a mudslide of emotion. I was in agony, drowning, wailing between breaths. A mother being forced to give up her child, one that wasn't conceived yet but still impossible to let go of. I climbed upstairs to get away from him. Standing no longer seemed stable and I ended up on the floor, coiled in between our laundry baskets, clinging to the grey woven fabric. One for whites, the other for colours, both spilling over with our dirty laundry. He tried to hug me, but I scuttled away, protecting myself. I couldn't be close to someone who was stamping on my heart like this, strangling our future.

'I feel so bad,' he said, pacing around our bedroom. 'Like I've committed a crime or something.'

'Then why are you doing it?' I roared. 'Do you understand how traumatic this is?'

He nodded. He said he was going on another walk and to call someone on the phone, I didn't ask who. I don't know what advice he was being given, but I can only imagine that any of his close friends or family were agreeing that he should not have a baby with someone he no longer wanted to have a baby with. Solid advice for anyone. But I was worried he was obscuring the truth, not telling them the full story to make his actions sound less serious. I wanted them to know the facts: the months of trying, the thousands of pounds' worth of private tests, the signed paperwork, the negative pregnancy tests, the ovulation strips, the mood-altering hormones, the needles in my belly, my diagnosis, my family's story. I wanted them to know that it was too late to change our minds. But most of all, I wanted them to know about the millions of moments before now when he could have mentioned how he was feeling. The car journeys, the endless walks, the fertility clinic waiting rooms.

I found his mum's number on my phone and started writing her a message.

Hi, sorry to contact you but

Perhaps she would be on my side? Maybe she could sway him back? Perhaps she could help us figure this out.

I don't know what James has told you

I typed out words but everything felt inadequate. What could she possibly say? She was his mum, she would always be on his side. I deleted the message. We were adults; it felt wrong to get his parents involved. And anyway, he was probably on the phone to them already.

I composed myself enough to call my mum. She answered and told me they were on their way to a friend's seventieth birthday party. Was it anything important? she asked. No, I replied, not wanting to gatecrash their evening. Just a catch-up, I'll call you tomorrow instead.

But I needed someone to talk to. Who else could understand? Who else could appreciate how unbearably late in the IVF process it was for someone to change their mind? I called my friend Alice. Alice was seven months pregnant with her own IVF baby and we'd been supporting each other through our respective fertility journeys. We'd stayed good friends since university and, as our friends reproduced around us, we had bonded in more recent years over our shared desire (and failure) to have our own children. IVF had worked first time for Alice and her husband, which was wonderful, though it had not been an easy road getting there.

'Oh my god, Bex,' she said. 'I can't believe he's doing this.'

'I know.' I paused and tried to breathe properly. 'It's like leaving someone at the altar on their wedding day.'

'I think it's worse than that,' she said. 'I don't think you can come back from something like this. It's such a breach of trust.'

Of course we can, I thought. We have to.

'Maybe we can just delay it all,' I said.

'But even if you do, it's such a horrendous thing to do to you.'

'I know.'

'And how do you know it won't happen again?'

'I know,' I sighed with my whole, heavy body.

I suddenly remembered that my friends were visiting for the weekend and would be arriving into Leeds train station soon. I felt a pang of anger that James had put me in this position, not broaching this conversation earlier in the day, before they boarded their train and travelled two hundred miles north. It wasn't fair for them to be walking into this.

I pulled myself together and got in the car to collect Lucy and Paul from the station. James asked if he should come with me, but I said no. I needed to figure out what I was going to say and I didn't want to start crying again in the car. But how to be a good hostess in a hurricane? I wondered if I could just pretend nothing had happened, but I've known Lucy since I was eleven years old; we have supported each other through the mistakes and messes of our lives for twenty years. She is one of the least judgemental people I know – a rare and valuable quality – and we have always been able to trust each other with the most unedited versions of ourselves. And she knew James too; the three of us had been on holiday together the year before. I needed her advice.

When Lucy and Paul got in the car and asked how I was, I told them. Paul looked a little bewildered and I was embarrassed that someone I didn't know was seeing me in such a crisis. I knew their own conversations about having children were fragile. No doubt witnessing my ordeal wasn't instilling them with confidence. But they were both kind and understanding and just very sorry it was happening. I offered them some options for the weekend: to go back to London, to spend the weekend just with me, or to explore the city on their own. They said they would do whatever I wanted; fun things to keep me distracted or give me space if I needed.

When we arrived back at the house it was time to do my evening IVF injection. I wondered if I should even still do it.

But I had come this far, I knew it would be crazy to cut the medication short and not at least try and salvage the eggs I had so carefully been incubating. Plus, James might change his mind.

After Lucy and Paul went to their room, James and I talked in bed and cried some more. I tried to fall asleep, but I couldn't. My brain was somersaulting, trying to make sense of how we'd got here; there was so much I didn't understand. James had deliberately caught the bouquet for us at my sister's wedding less than a month before. We'd had a wonderful holiday in France with his family the week before that. I couldn't comprehend how things had changed so quickly. The previous weekend we had stumbled across a car boot sale and giggled as we foraged together, buying a yoga mat, a framed portrait of a ginger cat and a metal colander with heart-shaped holes. I bought the colander because ours was plastic and a fertility book I'd read advised against plastic kitchen utensils. Now my whole world felt like that colander: porous and slipping through my fingers, through heart-shaped holes.

I wandered downstairs and sat on the steps outside our house wearing just a T-shirt, pants and no shoes. I sobbed quietly so the neighbours wouldn't hear. Life felt unbearable.

When James and I were falling in love, the world was falling apart. We spent the long days of lockdown at our parents' houses at different ends of the country, calling, messaging and emailing each other from our bedrooms. We were in our late twenties, but it felt like we were teenagers again. The whole world had come to a stop, literally, the way it always seems to when you are falling in love. James began a routine of reading me a poem by voice note before bed every night and I loved listening to them when I awoke in the morning.

One of the first poems he read to me was 'Night of Sleepless Love' by Federico García Lorca.

Night above us with the full moon,
I began to weep, while you laughed.
Your disdain was a god and my lament,
A momentary shackled dove.

Night below us. A crystal of sorrow,
You cried for the deepening distance.
My pain a cluster of agonies
Upon your weak heart of sand.

Dawn joined our bodies on the bed,
Our mouths pressed to the frozen stream
drinking the endless blood we shed.

And through the shutters came the sun
And the coral of life unfurled its branches.

When he wrote this poem, Lorca was lovesick and heartbroken. He was a close friend (and likely a lover) of Salvador Dalí. They were each other's muses, but beyond that we cannot be sure. Whether the love was unrequited or just unconsummated, biographers disagree, though homosexuality's illegality at the time has no doubt muddied the water for historians. After Lorca was murdered in 1936, Dalí seemed to be haunted for decades by what could have been.

When we go through dark nights of the soul in our relationships, we do not know if they will change the course of our lives or not. They can feel so life-shattering in the moment, but only hindsight reveals if they are. These junctures – an argument, a text message, a change of heart – can dictate our futures. They can shape our extended families and who our future children are, or whether we have them. I often think of the scene in *Back to the Future* when Marty McFly watches everyone slowly fade away in his family photograph as he realises his actions are jeopardising his own existence in the future. There are moments in life that can feel like that, literally altering our future family portraits. That weekend with James was one of them. I did not know if it would make or break us, but I knew something would change.

I got back into bed around 4 a.m. and managed a few hours of sleep. I woke to find that James had risen early, bought fresh pastries and berries from the local deli and was in the kitchen making coffee for everyone. He was always a good host. For a minute I dared to feel hopeful, but when we spoke I realised that this breakfast was just a peace offering. He had not changed his mind, he said. I had no appetite. While everyone else enjoyed breakfast, I went upstairs and wrote a letter on my laptop.

It's hard to look back at this letter now. I simply could not see a way of continuing with my life. I was in a state of shock, distressed that someone I loved so much could do this to me and devastated that my dream of having a child was being extinguished. I was also pumped full of artificial hormones from the fertility treatment; my mental state had been fragile for weeks. At that point it felt unsalvageable.

When I finished writing the letter, I walked outside to cry on the doorstep again, where no one could see me. I could hear Lucy, Paul and James joking and laughing inside the house, behaving normally, like everything was fine. Like my life hadn't just capsized. Like I wasn't dying a few metres away. I wanted to scream.

I didn't blame Lucy and Paul; they were just being polite and trying to muddle through an awkward situation. But I hated James, I hated that he could be two people at once: charming and funny and kind to them but confusing and reckless to me. Eventually he came outside to see where I was. Through tears, I told him how painful it was to hear them all laughing, knowing that this was one of the worst days of my life. He said he was so sorry, they didn't mean to cause me more distress, that they all loved me. He wrapped his arms around me and I sank into his warm body. But the relief lasted only a few seconds. I told him about the letter. I told him to go upstairs, open my laptop and read it.

I wanted him to know how much I was hurting and how pointless my life seemed now. But I can only imagine that the letter pushed James further away, confirming his fears about my psychological state. I must have seemed so unstable to have written those things. My mental health had not been good for a few years. A stressful job, a chronic illness, a global pandemic and entering my thirties feeling so behind where I'd hoped to be in my personal life, not to mention the secret I was keeping from my family, still gnawing away at me. All these ingredients, each enough on their own to curdle the core of a person, had whipped me up into an anxious state of depression, distrust and, at times, despair. Infertility was just the cherry on top.

My determination and desire to be a mother were so important, so crucial to my being, that ironically I probably now seemed unfit to be one. The message was clear: any future I felt worth living was dependent on James. My future happiness was wrapped around having a family with him and without that nothing else seemed worth sticking around for. That's a lot of pressure for a partner.

But my friends were visiting, so we would have to talk again properly when they left the next day. I put on a brave face and a floaty dress and we continued with our original Saturday plans, minus James. The three of us caught a bus into town and visited a bakery, a vintage shop and a cocktail bar. The distractions were good and I only cried a couple of times during the day, disguised by sweat due to the unseasonable September heatwave. Mum messaged to ask if it was a good time for her to call back. I replied telling her that I was out with friends and hinted that James was having second-thoughts about the IVF. She sent back the emoji that looks like Munch's *The Scream*.

James joined us in the evening for a drink at a riverside bar. We went for a meal and everything felt pretty normal again. We were just four young people on a double date eating delicious Indian food and having a good time. James and I loved each other. We would get past this blip.

A few hours later we arrived home and had a chance to talk privately again. After such a lovely evening I dared to feel optimistic, but he confirmed, again, that he had not changed his mind. It winded me.

'I need to call my mum,' I said.

'That's probably a good idea,' he replied.

I told him to leave the house. I couldn't spend another night in the same bed as him; I was too exhausted to not sleep again. He grabbed a few things and walked out the door. It was late so he called friends for a sofa to stay on, but no one picked up, so he headed towards a B&B down the road. I stabbed my belly with the evening IVF injection then called my mum.

'Hi darling, is everything okay?'

But I couldn't form any words, I just howled into the phone; a guttural roar of despair.

'I'll come over right now,' she said. I heard Dad mumble in the background. 'Oh, I've had a glass of wine, but I'll be okay to drive, I'll see you soon. I love you.'

She jumped in the car and drove the ninety minutes north to my house. While Lucy and Paul were asleep in the room next door, Mum stayed up listening and comforting me in bed for hours as I cried and tried to make sense of what was happening. Around midnight, I was shattered and suggested we go to sleep. Mum politely asked if I would mind if she went downstairs to eat a boxed salad she had brought with her. I had called her just as she and Dad were about to tuck into their dinner.

'Oh my goodness,' I said. 'Of course, you must be starving. I'm so sorry.'

The next morning I had an appointment with the fertility clinic to check how my follicles were developing. Mum came with me and we left Lucy and Paul to wander around the suburbs of Leeds on their own. As we walked through the automatic doors of the tired teaching hospital, I felt the long corridors and stairwells shrinking around us. The clinic reception was shiny and bright; newer than the rest of the hospital, or at least better kept, being partially privately funded. The waiting room had felt like a sanctuary of hope for months; I always looked forward to the appointments, even the ones involving blood or catheters. But that morning I felt like a child walking towards the headteacher's office, not sure if I was in trouble or not. As the nurse called me through, I asked if it was okay to bring my mum in with me.

'Of course,' said the nurse, a lady with bright pink hair and a warm smile. A friendly nurse makes all the difference, I thought, especially on days like this.

'How have you been finding the medication?' she asked.

'The injections have been fine, but the pills made me feel awful,' I said. 'I kept bursting into tears all the time, even at work.'

'Oh yes, everyone says that,' she said, nodding.

And we're just expected to endure it, I thought. Why did wanting a baby mean I had to go slightly insane first? It got me wondering if my change in mood had been responsible for James's change of heart. Did he worry that these mood swings would come back again in pregnancy, post-birth or the difficult early years of child-rearing? It felt like another injustice of infertility. Some of us have no choice but to conceive like this, in the turbulence of synthetic hormones.

I lay down on the bed and the nurse began a transvaginal ultrasound scan of my ovaries.

'You have lots of nice, big, juicy follicles,' she said, after a few minutes of manoeuvring the large wand.

I was relieved that the eggs were developing well; some good news finally. She did not ask about my partner, or if I had one.

'You went through all this thirty years ago, didn't you?' I said as I looked over at Mum who was sitting behind the blue curtain. 'Has it changed much?'

'Oh, you had IVF too?' the nurse asked, smiling.

'Yeah,' Mum replied. 'I think the odds are better now – back then they only gave me a 7 per cent chance of it working.'

'Wow, that's amazing,' the nurse said. 'An IVF baby having an IVF baby!'

But I didn't know if I was going to have a baby. Or even the option to have a baby. As it stood, all I had were follicles. Still, I was trying to stay positive. I had done so much to get to this point, I didn't want these eggs to go to waste. But the NHS does not pay for single women to freeze their eggs; they will only fund IVF if a partner is involved. I was in a stalemate.

'Because you've got some follicles measuring really big, it's likely the consultant will want you to take your trigger shot tonight,' the nurse said. 'Which means the egg retrieval should take place on Tuesday morning.'

The trigger shot was the final injection, encouraging the eggs to mature so they would be perfectly ripe for retrieval. For this part, timing is imperative; the injection needs to be done precisely thirty-six hours before the scheduled egg collection.

After the appointment, Mum and I found a place to eat nearby and discussed what I should do regarding James. Putting our future as a couple aside, we agreed that the practicalities of the IVF were the most important thing to decide on right now. I drove us home and a couple of hours later the clinic called to confirm that I needed to do my trigger shot just after midnight that evening. I texted James and asked him to meet me at the house. He said he'd just been for a run, was about to shower at the B&B and would head over after. When he arrived Mum was in the kitchen, and they said hello as if everything was normal. Mum offered to go for a walk to give us some space, but I said we'd go out instead. In the beating September sun, we wandered over to our local park and sat on the grass. I told him about the update from the fertility clinic. There were four options now, I explained.

'Number one, we carry on with the IVF as planned. You turn up on Tuesday and give your sperm while they collect my eggs and we go ahead with it all.'

'I'm sorry, but I'm not going to do that,' he said.

'Number two,' I continued, 'you turn up on Tuesday, provide your sample, they fertilise the eggs and then freeze the embryos.' I brightened my tone of voice to make him feel like this was the best option. 'That way we can postpone the IVF for as long as we want: six months or a year, and do the embryo transfer later on, when you're ready.'

It was the option I was hoping he would agree to. Buy more time, put our future on ice.

'It's a much better option than just freezing my eggs,' I said. 'Because embryos are far more likely to stay intact and survive the thawing process.'

James looked down. I could feel my heart beat in my throat.

'Bex, I'm sorry, but I've made up my mind. I'm not going to give a sample.'

I felt sick. He sounded so dogged and assertive. *Be firm with her*, I imagined his friends and family telling him. *You've made your decision.*

'The third option is I go to the egg collection on Tuesday and freeze my eggs, hoping they agree to that and don't invoice me for the thousands of pounds of medication I've used.'

'I think you should try and do that,' he said.

I struggled to look at him and twiddled some grass in between my fingers.

'The final option is I cancel the appointment, or they don't agree to freeze the eggs and everything is wasted.'

'Sorry, Bex, but I'm not going to be there on Tuesday.'

My heart broke again. I felt foolish for thinking this conversation might change his mind, and even more foolish for thinking I could finally have something I had wanted for so long. Not even a child, just a *chance* at having one, a one in three chance. All the percentages and predictions and possibilities were disintegrating now; it was all meaningless.

'But,' I said in one last, pathetic push, 'the fertility clinic doesn't let patients leave the hospital on their own, because of the sedation.'

I was hoping he might offer to give me a lift there and back; surely it was the least he could do in the circumstances? And if he was there in person, there was still a small chance; he might change his mind and surprise me.

'I'm sorry, I can't. I've got a busy schedule that day,' he said. 'I need to be in Nottingham to help with some interviews.'

Are you fucking kidding me, I thought. We were working on the same series and I knew it wasn't crucial that he was at those interviews. We both knew no one would mind if he told our bosses that he had to take me to hospital instead. It felt like another blow. As if fertility treatment wasn't already a woman's burden, he was forcing me to turn up to our appointment alone, explain why we were abandoning our round of IVF and then arrange my own transport home.

As we walked back to the house it became clearer that James was contemplating our entire relationship, not just the prospect of children. One of my deepest wishes is that he'd have understood the significance of separating the two, rather than muddling them up into one knotty atrocious nightmare. James had been by my side through the aftermath of my own family discovery, supported me when I told my siblings the truth and then, most painfully, my dad. He had witnessed the appalling symptoms of my endometriosis on a weekly basis and knew that having children was something doctors advised I do as soon as possible. It was something we had talked about since the week we met. And yet here he was, breaking up with me in the middle of an IVF cycle we had both signed up for. I couldn't think of a more brutal way to break someone's heart, especially mine.

Later that day James caught a train to London to stay with a friend. He said he needed some headspace for a few days. A few hours later, Mum headed home, leaving me on my own for the first time all weekend. She had offered to stay until Tuesday for the egg collection, but I knew she had things to do and didn't want to disrupt her week any further. She agreed to come back early on Tuesday morning to take me to the hospital. Logistically, I needed someone to take me but also knew how hard it would be to explain my change of circumstances to the staff. I might not be able to talk through my tears; I needed her to help me advocate for myself, to persuade them to agree to freeze my eggs. Her potential grandchildren.

I was exhausted but had to stay up past midnight to do the trigger shot. James had been by my side during all the other injections, but this time I was on my own. I have never felt so deeply alone in all my life than when I stuck that final needle into my belly. It was supposed to be an injection of hope but it felt like an untethering; an act of deep surrender into an unknown future.

Patient

Definition

1. A person receiving medical treatment
2. Having patience

We were in the editing stage of the hospital series we'd filmed over the summer, working with a team of around thirty others. I mostly worked from home, as did James, but two or three times a week we would drive two hours into the centre of Manchester to work in the office. Monday morning arrived and I needed to be in the office for some meetings. I had only told one colleague about the IVF treatment: my editor, Sean, a lovely Scouse man in his late twenties. He was the person I worked most closely with and I felt he should know in advance if I had to pop out for a last-minute hospital appointment.

On the drive in that morning I couldn't stop crying, my tears blurring the road. I imagined deliberately crashing my car on the motorway, contemplating how I could do it without hurting anyone else.

Just get through today, I thought, as I walked into the edit suite, determined not to mention what had happened.

'How was your weekend?' Sean asked.

Before I could say anything, tears started gushing out of me. How stupid to think that I could contain it. I had no choice but to tell him. Sean walked over and gave me a long hug. He had witnessed the emotional maelstrom of the previous weeks, as the high dose of hormones left my emotions teetering at all times. I really wasn't the type to cry at work, or at all, so I was embarrassed by how many times Sean had already seen me cry in just a few weeks, and now this. He looked confused and sad for me. He knew James; I'd introduced them and they got on well, even texting about cricket and football sometimes. As James's desk – just outside our edit suite – remained noticeably empty, I muddled through the day, trying to focus on our episode. I didn't want to let Sean and the wider team down.

Somehow I got through the meetings and avoided any conversations with colleagues about James. For the first time in my career I was running two edits at once, so I also had another episode to manage at the same time. It should have been a brilliant step forward for my career, but instead I was living in a nightmare. How could I possibly manage the intense workload alongside such overwhelming emotion? I didn't know how I would get through the week, never mind the remaining month of my contract.

I didn't feel I could tell my bosses about what had happened. It felt deeply unprofessional to bother them with the intricacies of our relationship and I didn't want them to think badly of James. I loved him. If we rekindled in a few days I would regret having said anything. So I pretended everything was fine and requested a day of leave for an unspecified 'medical procedure' the following day.

The next morning I woke up early and gathered my things for a day in hospital. I hoped James would send me a message. In spite of everything, it was still a relatively risky procedure. Under heavy sedation the doctors would insert a giant needle through my cervix and pierce both my ovaries in turn, sucking eggs from as many tiny follicles as they could. There was a small risk of accidentally puncturing other organs, infection and a scary side effect called ovarian hyperstimulation syndrome, which can be fatal. I kept checking my phone; still no text. I decided to message him instead.

> Hope your interviews go well today x

> **Thanks Bex, I hope today goes well and I hope your mum is with you. I'm sorry from the bottom of my heart that I'm not there with you.**

It was sinking in. He was not going to turn up. I would not have his baby or embryos or even the courtesy of a lift to the hospital. I felt lucky to even get a text back.

Mum knocked on the door and we climbed into her car. When we arrived at the hospital, I was nervous. I had been practising pretend conversations in my head, trying to find the right words to explain to the staff what had happened and why my partner was not there with me.

'Hi, it's Rebecca Coxon,' I said to the receptionist. 'I'm here for my egg retrieval.'

'Hello, yes, if you just head through those doors and follow them round to the other waiting room,' she replied.

'Thank you. Also, I wondered if . . .' I paused. 'If I could talk to a doctor or nurse about something. Something about my partner.'

'Yes, if you flag down a nurse while you're in there, they can help you.'

'Thank you.'

Mum and I sat in the waiting room, clinical and bare, with just a water dispenser to look at. Mercifully we were the only ones there; I didn't need an audience for this conversation or to be around happy couples trying to conceive together. Eventually a nurse walked past.

'Excuse me,' I said, my voice shaking. Mum put her hand on

my back. 'I'm here for an egg retrieval today, for IVF. But erm, well, my partner has told me he's not going to show up.'

'Oh. Okay,' she replied.

'So I wondered if it's possible to still go ahead and freeze my eggs? I've taken all the medications and the trigger shot at the right time. Obviously I don't want to waste it all.'

'Right, okay. I'm sure that'll be fine. There might be some paperwork to sign, but I'll need to just check with the doctor first.'

'Of course. Thank you.' The nurse walked away and I turned to Mum.

'At least I didn't cry,' I said.

'You did really well,' she said.

I got changed into my hospital gown and was allocated a bay and a bed to lie on. Ten minutes later, a woman in her forties peered round the curtain.

'Hello, is it Rebecca?'

'Yes.'

'I'm the consultant on the ward today, and my colleague tells me there's been an issue with your partner, is that right?'

'Yeah.' I took a deep breath. 'He told me he isn't going to turn up today to do the sample.'

'I'm really sorry to hear that,' she said, her face full of compassion and concern, a look I was familiar with in my job. It was the kind of expression we zoomed in on with our cameras, adding poignant music to milk the jeopardy. But this time it was for my benefit, I was the patient with the bad news. I was the one being comforted by a doctor.

'Do you think he's likely to come in later?' she continued. 'Or has he changed his mind about the IVF completely?'

'I don't know. I'm really confused about it all,' I said. 'All I know is that he's definitely not coming in today. And I'm just really hoping you can still collect my eggs.'

'Okay, well the good news is that, yes, we can still go ahead with the egg collection, that's fine. It'll just be a case of you paying for storage of the eggs because the NHS does not fund women on their own.'

I nodded. It was not the first time they had encountered an issue with collecting a sperm sample on the day of an egg retrieval, she told me, though the other instances sounded more to do with men having stage fright than deserting their partners.

'If your partner does come back on board in the future then we can continue with the IVF for free, but if you decide to continue the process on your own then you would have to self-fund the remainder of the treatment.'

'Yes, I understand. Thank you.'

Several hours later I was wheeled into the operating room and met with warm smiles from six women in scrubs and facemasks. They introduced themselves individually and I felt like I was in safe hands.

'You're an all-female team,' I smiled. 'That's amazing.'

'Yep, you've got the dream team on today!' the embryologist said.

I was put to sleep and woke up twenty minutes later, as they were collecting the final egg.

'Another one, number six,' I heard someone say while half-conscious.

In a normal round of IVF, the eggs would be placed in a Petri dish, mixed with the partner's sperm and left in an incubator overnight. For me, though, it was IVF without the F. There would be no hot date; my eggs had been stood up. Instead they were frozen in a tank of liquid nitrogen. For how long, I did not know.

A few hours later the clinic emailed me photos of six adorable circles. Snapshots of single cells not yet ensouled. Potential people. Specks of hope. But only half the ingredients.

Mum drove us home and cooked pasta as I lay on the sofa while the anaesthetic wore off. I scrolled through options on the

TV and settled on a documentary about a Swedish artist neither of us had heard of called Hilma af Klint, an abstract painter who was shunned to obscurity. When over a thousand of her paintings were discovered in 1986, forty years after her death, art historians were forced to rewrite history. Despite clear evidence that af Klint's work had been years ahead of her male counterparts Mondrian, Malevich and Kandinsky – the 'founding fathers' of abstraction – many historians refused to acknowledge her. She was an unwelcome disruption to the status quo.

At first her paintings appear simple; colourful, bold geometric shapes, but be patient and you'll find yourself absorbed in their intricate patterns, organic forms and superb spirals remarkably similar to the double helix of DNA, then not yet discovered. Af Klint was a mystic, a conduit – painting things we could not yet see or understand – at a time when electromagnetic waves, subatomic particles and radiation were only on the periphery of human understanding.

'The Ten Largest', her most famous series, follows a progression through human life from 'childhood', 'youth', 'adulthood' into 'old age'. In them, I see conception: eggs, sperm, fertilisation, cells dividing, harmony, chance, energy, life.

Today af Klint has at last been acknowledged as a pioneer of abstract art, but aside from misogyny in the art world, there is another reason why her paintings were hidden for so long; she requested they not be seen until twenty years after her death because she feared they would not be understood by the people of her time. Sometimes society stumbles, we must be patient.

After the documentary Mum left and I geared myself up for going back to work the next day. In the past I have found work to be a good distraction from heartbreak, but when the person who breaks your heart is a colleague, it feels like there is no escape. Except that James stopped coming into the office. I had no idea where he was or when he was going to come back up north. I messaged him, but he replied only occasionally, ignoring my questions for days at a time. When he did reply, his messages were often cryptic and torturously vague. He needed 'space', he kept saying, but I didn't know what that meant or for how long. I didn't know if we were still together or not and it felt humiliating.

One of our colleagues, Holly, texted me regularly to 'check in' and see how I was doing. Whenever we were both in the office, she invited me for lunch. I was so grateful for these gestures. Years before, I had worked for the production company that Holly runs with her wife, Kate. They have two daughters, one conceived with a sperm donor and another who is adopted, so Holly knew the strains of fertility treatment and creating a family more than most and was aghast that I had been left in this situation. She was one of the only people I felt I could talk to honestly about everything.

Eventually, James gave me a date he planned to return to Leeds, but then changed his mind at the last minute, which was exasperating. He did this several more times. Later I found out that he had asked our manager for some sort of compassionate leave and was granted permission to spend a week in the countryside with his family. Meanwhile I continued to commute into the office alone.

I was furious, but still in love with him, emotionally to-ing and fro-ing between trying to salvage our relationship and the sharp, intense frustration at his silence and utter nebulousness. Every time my rage erupted over text, he used it as evidence of why we shouldn't be together. He told me he couldn't be with someone who was so 'hot and cold'. I tried to muzzle my emotions, but it felt impossible. He had ripped up our future and I didn't know what to do. Every attempt to reconcile was met with silence or him needing more 'space'. I felt desperate and completely lost.

After several weeks, I needed an answer. Hanging on to any hope was driving me insane and destroying my dignity. Finally he called me. It was the weekend and rather than stew in despair at home, I had forced myself to go to a local poetry festival that I'd originally booked us both tickets for. I was sitting in the booth of a bar, waiting for the next event to start when my phone rang.

'How's the festival?' he asked.

'You would have loved it,' I said. 'Simon Armitage just hosted a panel about climate change and it was brilliant. Really interesting.'

'That sounds wonderful. I'm sorry I can't be there.'

'Can you just tell me if it's over between us?' I asked, feeling sick. 'Please just be honest. It's been weeks, I just need to know now.'

'I needed space, Bex,' he said for the hundredth time. 'If you're pushing me for an answer right now . . .' he said, then paused. He wanted me to force him into it, to avoid being the bad guy.

'This is unfair, James, I need an answer.'

'Then, yes,' he replied. 'I guess I would have to say it's over.'

Everything inside me drained.

'Thank you for actually saying it,' I said, despondent and pathetic. I hung up and melted into tears, covering my face while the bar staff pretended not to notice. After composing myself in the bathroom, I walked into the next poetry session, suddenly determined not to let him ruin any more of my plans. But it was impossible to absorb the beauty of anything right now. I needed to get home and drown in peace. I left before it started.

A week later James hired a van without telling me and removed his things from our house while I was at work. Walking into our home after that – half of it removed – felt like walking through a guillotine. The flowers James had bought me the day he abandoned the IVF were still in a vase, limp and half-alive. I couldn't believe they had outlasted our relationship. Who buys flowers for someone they are about to break up with? Every time I caught sight of them on the windowsill I felt queasy and confused, but couldn't bring myself to throw them away. They were the last thing I had of him; evidence that he existed at all, and that he once liked me enough to buy me flowers. I had no idea that the photograph of me holding them outside the porch that day – so hopeful and looking forward to being a mother – would be the last he ever took of me.

I believe anyone should be allowed to leave a relationship whenever they want, and that just wanting to leave is enough of a reason. Nobody should feel trapped. But the way you leave is important. The timing is important and the aftermath is important. Why get someone's hopes up and then so cruelly snatch them away? I will never understand why James chose our ending to be wrapped up in the dashing of my deepest hopes. I forgive him for leaving – it's what he needed to do – but that our break-up story, our swan song, the last moments of our relationship, are so painfully entwined with my infertility feels unforgivable.

Over the following weeks I felt broken open. I had lost my partner, my in-laws and my future children overnight. I learned that love is not a permanent marker, it can be wiped out in an instant. Yet I couldn't help but wonder: if we'd gotten pregnant naturally in the year we were trying, would we still be together? Or would he have deserted me still, and the baby too? I blamed myself. My body and my inability to get pregnant had done this. We both knew people for whom parenthood had been unplanned. You stepped up to the plate if it happened like that, there was no time to think and question. It was thrust upon you and you did the right thing. But not for people like me. Infertility gives you time to run away.

There would be no secrets or surprises any more. No announcements, no baby on the way. When I told friends what had happened, I watched their faces drop in shock. Some had been expecting me to tell them I was pregnant, but I had to say no, we didn't even get that far. He left me in the middle of IVF. It felt shocking to say it out loud every time. There was nothing left to hide behind now, no shell to contain my entrails. Family and friends rallied round, inviting me on dog walks, pub crawls, fondue nights and dance classes. I had never felt so popular, but each day was a monumental struggle.

James had always been the main cook in our relationship, and I, the washer-up. When he left, I went from eating the most nutritious meals we could muster to improve our chances at IVF, to not eating much at all. I lost weight. My clothes loosened at a time I'd hoped they would be getting tighter. Instead of buying maternity clothes I was downsizing all my jeans to stop them from falling down. There was no baby, just less of me. I had always wanted to be this skinny, I thought, but life doesn't always grant us the things we want when we want them. I would much rather have had a baby in my belly instead.

On the loneliest nights I would scour the internet for stories of people who'd had the same thing happen to them, but I couldn't find any. Not a single story like mine on any forum, newspaper or blog. Had it never happened before? Or was it just too shameful to write about?

I came back to the articles by Lena Dunham and her experience of trying to have a baby after a hysterectomy.

'I was forced to admit just how much of it was about finishing what I started,' she wrote. 'I tried to have a child. Along the way, my body broke. My relationship did, too. In the process – because of it? – I became a functional junkie. I had lost my way ... Each step took the process further from my body, my family, my reality.'

My relationship had also broken down as I navigated the intense process of trying to start a family with a broken body. I realised that all along I had been staring at a map on my own while James stood behind me secretly trying to navigate a way out. I hadn't noticed, or I'd refused to acknowledge it. He didn't want a child yet; he had just gone along with everything to avoid upsetting me. In the end it badly hurt us both.

Some weeks later, I was told the story of a friend of a friend. She was in a same-sex relationship and they were undergoing IVF, but her partner broke up with her in the middle of the process too.

So it *had* happened before. I felt relief and empathy. She still had a baby though, they said. She used the donor sperm they had bought and forged ahead on her own. But I didn't have any sperm. The story was offered as a slice of hope, but it made me feel empty. She's now raising the child as a single parent and seems very happy, they said. That's good to know, I replied, feeling a million miles away from that scenario myself. But at the age of thirty-two, newly single, with low ovarian reserve and worsening endometriosis, I realised that donor sperm might be my only realistic option for having a child. It felt like my life was coming full circle.

Six weeks after the break-up, Sophie was diagnosed with a brain tumour. In the months leading up to her surgery, the wombies – Zoe, Ruth and I – rallied round her. We listened, we hugged, we laughed and we watched Disney films, but between the smiles Sophie was, understandably, terrified. Her worst nightmare was coming true. After the surgery she would be placed on the high-dependency unit, or, if things didn't go to plan, the intensive care unit. As an intensive care nurse herself, Sophie knew what that meant. She knew how quickly life could slip through one's fingers. She knew about the risk of infections and blood clots, of strokes and comas, the side effects of major surgery. She saw it every day – she taught students how to care for these patients – and now she was going to be one of them.

The tectonic plates of my life were shifting again and my sense of reality, which I had tried to piece back together since the family secret, felt scrambled once more. I couldn't handle any more bad news. Sophie had been treating children with brain tumours one day and was having brain surgery herself the next. Everything could change in an instant. The universe does not care about your plans. It's all a mirage.

Single

Definition

1. Only one
2. Not married or in a relationship
3. An individual person or thing

My dad didn't know we were going through IVF because I wanted the pregnancy announcement to be a surprise. I couldn't face telling him what had happened so I asked Mum to. A few days later, we spoke on the phone.

'What did Dad say?' I asked.

'He said he could understand it from James's perspective,' she replied.

I didn't know whether to laugh or cry.

'Oh,' I said, 'that doesn't feel good to hear. He's basically saying he understands why someone wouldn't want to have children with me.'

It was the first conclusion my brain came up with. My relationship with James had burned holes in my self-esteem, but the break-up had set it on fire.

'I think he means,' she said, 'that he can understand it from a man's perspective. Why he left when he did.'

I didn't know how these comments were supposed to make me feel, but in the moment I felt utterly dejected, like Dad was taking James's side, or some sort of universal male angle. From a man's perspective, why was this all so difficult? Why do men avoid taking responsibility for their actions? Why do they so often abandon their partners before, during or after pregnancy? Why, when hard conversations need to be had, do they suddenly evaporate into thin air? And why do we not only tolerate it as a society but almost *expect* it from men?

It's a lonely place to be, a woman who is mad at men. I knew that most men were not like this, but when the two closest to me – my father and my partner – seemed to agree that abandoning me was the right thing to do, I felt hurt.

When I spoke to Mum about this conversation later, she admitted she'd relayed it badly and that I had misunderstood what Dad meant. Although the timing was terrible, Dad was just relieved that we'd broken up *before* I'd gotten pregnant. Did I wish James had shown up and allowed me a chance to have his children, even if he decided to leave me later on? Would that have been better than the position I was in? I didn't know. Only time and hindsight would tell. All I knew was that I would have loved that summer baby with all my heart.

'He said he would support you if you wanted to use a sperm donor,' Mum said.

'Oh.' I was taken aback. 'Really? He said that?'

'Yep. He wants you to be happy and he said he'd support you if that's what you decided to do. We both would, of course.'

I wasn't expecting her to say this, or at least not so soon after the break-up. It felt five steps ahead of where I was, but it had been on my mind. Part of me was still hoping James and I would get back together, while another part was, like them, wondering if it was too late to wait for another relationship. I also worried that my heart, once healed, could not risk going through something like this again.

I had always wondered how my parents would feel about me going it alone. They wanted me to have the safety and stability of a marriage, like them, but they also wanted me to be happy.

That day it felt like they were saying they thought I was capable of doing it on my own, that I didn't need someone else. And, more than that, my dad was telling me that using a sperm donor was okay, acceptable, not a problem. I think it was a way of him accepting it himself. We did it, you could do it too. And whatever happens, we'll be here for you.

As I reluctantly dipped my toe into the dating world again, after seven years' absence, I was alarmed and bewildered by what I found. At one point I had to call the police when someone started harassing me, so incensed that I'd politely declined to see him again after one date. Another time I had to report threatening messages to a dating app. Other people were kind, but there was no chemistry and I started to realise how rare a real connection was. It made a bleak time feel even bleaker.

I wasn't ready to go down the sperm donor route, but I figured there was no harm in looking, so I spent a few days trawling through sperm banks online. Some websites offered more information than others – beyond the basics of job, height, eye colour, ethnicity and hair colour – including photos of the donors as young children. Seeing these gorgeous little toddlers made me feel more broody. With some banks you could even listen to the donors' voices and some of them provided handwritten notes, which I found the most endearing.

> Dear Mother, parents,
>
> It would be an honour to be the chosen one to help you, for I believe that if you are reading this letter, it means that you possess a grand amount of love ready to be channelled into a child.

Once I started reading their letters, I couldn't stop. Some were serious, others were funny.

Hello there. First of all I really hope that you have not inherited my handwriting. Otherwise I hope that you are grateful for life and appreciate your surroundings.

Some offered their reasons for donating.

I have three really healthy, strong and talented children, and would like to pass it on to some who are not able to have children themselves.

Some included spelling mistakes and words crossed out, like a twelve-year-old's homework.

Hi. I am happy to be abel to help you get one of the biggest wishes in life ~~full~~fulfilled, I hope you become fantastic parents. Sincerely, Your Donor

Some were very short; others several pages long, sharing stories of their own upbringing or offering life advice.

Don't let the world or other people determine your worth.

Some felt like a personal pep talk, like they were rooting for us, for our families, for me.

Life is a beautiful thing. It is a confusing miracle that is hard to fully explain. Most times it is lovely and wonderful but it can also be hard and devastating. I have definitely experienced both parts. And most likely you will too.

These letters, from strangers to the mothers of their unborn children, felt healing to me. It was a distillation of the goodness in humans. In men.

After a few hours, I forced myself to shut my laptop, lest I start seriously considering one of them as the biological father of my child. Perhaps this one:

> Remember, it's a vast universe but you're a star in it. You can be anything you decide to be, it's your story to write. Let your heart guide you. And wherever you go, whatever you do ... always believe in the magic within you. Your journey is going to be an amazing one. And I'm cheering for you.

I thought about how different things had been for my parents. Today the choice is overwhelming. How do you choose between the profiles of eight hundred different men to be the genetic father of your child? Would it be based on appearance, personality, career? The way his voice sounds, his academic achievements, the sports he loves? Would his favourite food or music taste be what gave him an edge over dozens of others?

My parents did not have these choices. The decision was made for them and they were happy about it. They left the genetics of their children up to strangers and I understand why. If you know nothing about the donor it's easier to pretend they don't exist.

A few weeks after James and I broke up, my friend Ella messaged about meeting up. Even though she lived just a couple of miles away, we hadn't seen each other in a few weeks owing to busy summer schedules. The last time I'd seen her we were playing doubles on our local tennis courts: Ella and her boyfriend versus James and me. When she contacted me, I was a little embarrassed about telling her that James and I had broken up. But she got in first; she had broken up with her boyfriend too. I couldn't believe it.

I met Ella through TV work. We were paired up as producer and editor on a documentary series about the police. When you work with an editor you spend hundreds of hours in a room with them, so you get to know them pretty well. Very soon we realised how similar our lives were. We'd both lived in London for years before moving north during the pandemic. We met our partners around the same time and we'd both been trying to get pregnant for a while with no luck. We had visited our GPs in the same month and been referred to the same fertility clinic. And now we were both going through break-ups at the same time, neither of us any closer to starting the families we'd hoped for.

But that's when our paths diverged. I started dating again, while Ella purchased a vial of sperm online. I had six eggs on ice and, aged thirty-two, I thought I probably still had time to meet someone. Ella, on the other hand, was thirty-seven, with no frozen eggs and didn't want to waste time waiting for the right person or rush into doing it with someone she wasn't sure about.

As I had taken a break from television to start a postgraduate degree, we no longer worked together but, both newly single, became each other's go-to for invites. We went to burlesque classes, cinema screenings and for late-night swims. We enjoyed all the cuisines Leeds had to offer, from Afghani food to sourdough pizza, all the while discussing fertility and our possible futures.

Rather than choose a donor from one of the big sperm bank databases, Ella used a matching service provided by the local fertility clinic. After filling out a questionnaire, they sent her a donor's profile.

> As someone who wants to start my own family in the future, I realised that not everyone has the opportunity to do that without the help of other people. It makes me genuinely happy to do what seems like such a small gesture for such massive reward.

He seemed thoughtful, reflective and accomplished at a young age. Ella loved his profile and paid £1,200 for a vial of his sperm and many more thousands to have her eggs collected and fertilised with it. After undergoing the IVF process, she forwarded me a video that the clinic had recorded through a microscope of the cells dividing. My belly fluttered as I watched a single grey bubble burst into two, then four, then eight, then sixteen. It was new life – the stage of IVF I hadn't reached – and with the tap of her thumb she had sent it to me through the ether, like magic.

Five days later, the blastocyst – the earliest stage of an embryo – was transferred into Ella's womb. Two weeks later she took a pregnancy test.

It was negative.

In the UK there are more single parent families than ever before. More than a fifth of all children are living with a single parent, 90 per cent of whom are mothers. Despite this, many countries in Europe do not allow women to access IVF treatment on their own and in most countries that do, it must be entirely self-funded.

While many single parent families are the result of a relationship breakdown, in the western world the 'solo motherhood by choice' movement is growing. Whether the 'choice' element is entirely accurate in all cases, I'm not sure. From what I've heard and read it seems that many women would rather have a partner to share the time and cost of child-rearing, but have not found anyone willing or suitable to do it with during their short biological window. In any case, these days it's not uncommon for women to skip the dating part entirely and raise a family on their own. As I considered that route for myself, I wanted to speak to someone who had already done it. The first person who came to mind was Dorothy Byrne.

Byrne is one of the most impressive and high-profile women behind the scenes of British media over the last few decades. She was the head of news and current affairs at Channel 4 Television for seventeen years before becoming editor-at-large. Her television programmes have won everything from BAFTAs to Emmys and she has even been a guest on the BBC's *Desert Island Discs*.

She is an author, has several honorary doctorates and in 2021 was appointed president of Murray Edwards College at the University of Cambridge.

'I didn't choose not to have a baby,' Byrne told me. 'I just thought it would happen. I thought one day I'd meet the right person and I'd have children.' It was a Monday afternoon and we'd arranged to talk over a video call.

'I went out with journalists,' she continued, 'and travelled a lot for work, so life was always a bit disrupted.'

When Byrne was forty, she was moving house during a blizzard, heaving heavy boxes upstairs, when she noticed she was bleeding.

'One of my sisters is a doctor and I asked her, is this a miscarriage? And she said yes.' But Byrne didn't know she was pregnant and hadn't wanted to be. Nevertheless, it got her thinking.

'I spent a weekend asking myself: if I don't try to get pregnant, will I be sorry? And I thought yes, I'll be sorry if I don't try.'

Dorothy was born in Scotland, but her accent has softened, the result of moving to England when she was eight. Wearing a floral top and sitting in front of a watercolour painting, she is less intimidating than the last time I saw her, in a dimly lit meeting room at the headquarters of Channel 4.

Byrne decided to use a sperm donor, but kept it quiet.

'Do you ring people up and say, I'm going to have my legs waxed? No, you don't. You just go and do it. I did it all without telling anybody.'

Her matter-of-factness reminded me of the way my parents talked about their road to parenthood, as minimally and stoically as possible.

'How did you choose the donor?' I asked.

'They asked me what I wanted and I told them I hadn't really thought about it.'

It strikes me how much emphasis we put on finding the right romantic partner, but when it comes to the biological parent of our child, some of us, including my parents, are rather less picky. In the end, all Byrne suggested was that the donor be white and have a degree – so the child would fit in with her family – and not wear glasses, as she didn't and always thought it would be inconvenient to have to do so.

'And they said, is that it? I said, yeah, that's it.'

At the age of forty-four, after five rounds of artificial insemination, she was pregnant. At the time she was the editor of *The Big Story*, an ITV current affairs series.

'I just told people I was pregnant, I didn't tell them how I'd got pregnant. I thought I'm not answering all your questions, I'm just getting on with my pregnancy.'

The only person to be upset by the news, Byrne said, was her mother. 'But the person who really surprised me was my father. He wasn't shocked at all and said he'd always wanted me to have a baby.'

A friend accompanied her to the birth and Byrne paid to have her own room so she didn't have to look at other women with their partners. She called her daughter Hettie.

'My dad said it was the best thing I'd ever done and he played a fatherly role in Hettie's life until the day he died.'

In terms of dating or a social life, it wasn't easy. Sometimes Byrne would wake up on the sofa to find a note from a friend saying, 'I was talking to you but you fell asleep so I left.'

'I actually went back to work when Hettie was five and a half weeks old, or I wouldn't have had a job. Someone else would just have got the job, and that was very hard, but I could afford a full-time nanny.'

Finances are, of course, an important factor in being able to raise a child on your own. Byrne could afford the cost of fertility treatment as well as a nanny to help her look after her child, but believes that giving birth should not depend on your bank balance. On top of that is the impact that time away and daily caring duties can have on your career.

'I've met so many young women in TV,' she said, 'who say they'd like to have a baby now but they can't because it would disrupt their career, and that's a disgrace.'

I know plenty of women like this. In fact, I was so afraid of being one of them that it's something I've tried to pre-empt since the start of my working life. In my twenties I made a conscious effort to get a head start, assuming it would help my career in the longer term when I inevitably paused to have children. As a woman, becoming a director in a predominantly male world felt like my glass ceiling and I wanted to break it before I had a baby. I worked extra hours, rented camera equipment and shot and edited my own films in my spare time. I entered competitions and won independent funding from film festivals. For ten years I gave it my all, always thinking in the back of my mind that being a fully fledged director would make it much easier to get work when I returned from maternity leave, as well as set me up financially for a family. At the age of twenty-seven I was offered my first directing job for prime-time television. I developed and pitched the idea to Channel 4 and the person who commissioned it was Dorothy Byrne. For the next eighteen months I produced, directed and filmed a documentary about child drug runners and it was during that time that I discovered I was donor-conceived. Back then I had no idea that Byrne had a donor-conceived child herself.

In the 1990s, as Byrne settled into life as a new parent, the editor of a magazine asked her to write an article about having a donor baby. She agreed, but the Channel 4 press office insisted she write it anonymously.

'Can you believe that? They said it would undermine my reputation as a serious journalist if people knew I had a baby by donor sperm. I was really angry that they basically strong-armed me. I have no idea why I went along with it.'

Later on, in an interview with a different newspaper, Byrne

mentioned in passing that she had a donor-conceived child, but this time they published her name.

'After I came out, so to speak, I would get these phone calls from women I didn't know saying, oh hello, I'm Amelia, I work in BBC Features, can I come and have a coffee with you? And I'd think, ah, right, you want to have a baby.'

A few years ago, Byrne met one of these women at a lunch.

'She said, oh you don't remember me but I came to visit you saying I was thinking of having a baby by donor insemination, what do you think? And you said, it's great, do it. Then she showed me a photograph of a lovely little boy and said, this is my son, thanks to you.'

Many of the women who spoke to Byrne had been advised not to do it by other people in their lives.

'And I'd say, well what do they know? The only person whose views you should pay any attention to are your own and perhaps someone who's actually done it.'

Speaking to Byrne, I was buoyed by a sense of empowerment, but in 2021, she was criticised for doing the opposite. When she took on the role of president of Murray Edwards – one of the only remaining all-female colleges of Cambridge University – she said she would talk openly about her experiences with sexual harassment, consent and the controversial F-word. But even the mention of fertility caused outrage among some and her plans were criticised as 'patronising', 'infuriating' and 'pro-natalist'. Byrne was accused of reducing women to the biological role of motherhood. 'The 19th century called,' wrote one critic, 'and they want their curriculum back.'

But Byrne felt that society had 'swung too far one way', with girls being encouraged to 'get themselves a great education and have great careers' while neglecting to mention anything about fertility and its finiteness or the joys of having a family, *if* that's something they wished to do. Some even called her anti-feminist, which is ironic considering that she is a pioneer in a male-dominated industry and spent years commissioning documentaries about women's rights.

Byrne had not anticipated such a vicious backlash, proving her point about just how taboo the subject still is. I asked her about that time.

'It's absolutely not true that I believe you have to have a child to be happy,' she said. 'Nor if you want a baby did I say you have to do it early. I had a baby at forty-five. I was the head of news and current affairs and now I'm the president of a Cambridge college; I believe in women being successful, but I do also believe in women being informed.'

If we are teaching young people how to use contraception and avoid pregnancy, we should also teach them how to get pregnant when the time comes, Byrne argues. One in six people will be affected by infertility in their lifetime so it makes sense for reproduction – like any other aspect of health – to be included on the educational agenda and I wholeheartedly agree.

'I don't lecture my students, but I talk about it,' she said. 'I had a baby and I talk about it absolutely openly, because I talk about my whole life. I talk about how to overcome sexism, what to do if you're assaulted at work, misogyny. I talk about everything I learned in my life that I think is useful to know, and one of the things that's really useful to know is some of the facts about fertility because we're not taught them at school, and we don't know them. And then, once you know the facts, and if you're interested in having children and have checked out your own fertility, then do what you like. It's your own business. I don't give advice to people on what to do in life.'

One of the students in her college, Sharon Blass, wrote an article for *Varsity*, agreeing that these conversations needed to be had. 'As a woman, particularly in my male-dominated department, it sometimes feels almost anti-feminist to include having a family as one of my future ambitions.'

I also felt like this in my teens and twenties. As women, it feels like we have a duty to continue breaking boundaries and rewriting gender norms; how dare we aspire to raise a family and defy the generations before us who had fewer choices?

Like getting engaged, I thought that falling pregnant was something to be sprung on you unexpectedly one day, if you were lucky, and loved. For those on whom it cannot be sprung – because they are single or their partner refuses or they require some medical intervention – it can feel like breaking some kind of feminist code by simply raising the subject. For those who don't meet their partner until their mid to late thirties, or at all, it can be a shock to discover that the boat – enabling them to be genetically related to their child – has sailed. Byrne admits that while her personal story is seen as inspirational by some women, she thinks they should take away the opposite message: she left it far too late and nearly missed out.

I told Byrne that I think women are generally more informed these days. Adverts for fertility testing companies seem to be everywhere now and my friends in their late twenties and early thirties (who don't already have children) have started talking about egg freezing or when to start trying. But the conversation doesn't seem to happen with men. I have found that many men in their thirties haven't thought about kids at all: whether they want them or when. 'They've got no sense of a biological clock,' I said, 'and obviously, their clock is ticking a little slower than women's—'

'But it's ticking,' Byrne chimed in. 'I think there's a lot of selfishness in men. I know a number of women who were with men in their late thirties, and the men were going, oh, well, I'm not ready yet. And they stayed with those men and they ended up not having children. And on more than one occasion, the relationship split up and almost immediately the man went off with another woman and had a child with her. I think sometimes men say I'm not ready to have children, but what they really mean is, I'm not ready to have children with *you*. Well, it would be better if they said that.'

'Yeah,' I said, feeling both reassured and alarmed that this was not just a problem for me, or my generation.

'I think it's a big issue that isn't talked about enough,' Byrne continued. 'But in the end, a woman may have to choose between having a baby and her relationship. And she might decide to choose the relationship.'

I told her how I resented being put in this position myself, trying to nudge things forward before it was too late, only to watch both my relationship and the prospect of a baby fall off a cliff.

'I think at school we should say to boys, you need to be aware, you might be able to carry on, but think of the woman you're having a relationship with,' Byrne said. 'Schools should be talking about all this.'

Byrne also wants schools to talk about infertility. 'When you talk about fertility, you need to talk about infertility,' she said, 'because when a woman or a man discovers they're infertile, they can suffer the most terrible blow to their self-esteem because it's a secret shame. But if we talked about it at school, it wouldn't be.'

On the subject of shame, I asked Byrne how she broached being donor-conceived with her daughter.

'I used to tell her so often that she never had a moment that she didn't know. I mean, if you're a single mother, you can't cover it up in the same way, but I also made a decision very early on that if I covered anything up I would be implying to my child that I thought there was something shameful and embarrassing about her, and I didn't.'

It is this difference – between being told and finding out – where shame breeds, I realised. I was glad to hear someone speak so directly about this, the idea that keeping a secret in and of itself is a symptom of shame.

'At first, I didn't know how to say it, there were no books then,' Byrne said. 'So I explained how sex worked, and then I said, but that wasn't what I did, I had you in a different way. And [Hettie] looked confused, and I thought, this isn't working. So I said I went to a clinic and a nice man gave me his seed and they put it inside me and it grew into you with my egg. And I would tell her that every four months and she would say . . . oh, not that story again.'

When Hettie was older, to help her understand, Byrne took her to meet the fertility doctor at the clinic where she was conceived, which Hettie happened to pass on the way to school every day. Sometimes her fellow pupils would ask Hettie about her father.

'At first she told people her father was dead. Brilliant. Even children don't ask any more questions. Then she told people that her father lived in China. I mean, it was so clever,' Byrne said, beaming at the ingenuity. 'I did once have to go into the playground to berate a boy who said she came from outer space or something. And I always said to her, there'll be more women, there'll be more children.'

Unbeknown to them, there already was. One day one of the other mothers – from Hettie's class of just fourteen children – asked Bryne if she was going to the annual Donor Conception Network meeting. Byrne said she wasn't sure if she could make it that year.

'And I said, sorry, do you go? And she said, oh yes, my daughter is donor-conceived. I said to Hettie, I told you there were other people . . . all these years there's actually been another girl in your class.'

In terms of knowing who the donor is, Hettie is one of just 29,725 people in the UK who have no legal right to know their parentage. She was born between August 1991 and April 2005, a period in which records were kept but donors were granted anonymity. For individuals like Hettie, identifiable information about her donor does exist, she is just not allowed to see it.

'I feel very strongly that you cannot pass on a lack of a legal right,' Byrne told me. 'I didn't have the right to give up that right for her. It's her right. And I think it's scandalous that there's this small group of people who don't have the right to know who their parents are.'

It may sound like a unique scenario, but there is a precedent, Byrne tells me. In 1976 the Adoption Act gave adopted adults the right to obtain their original birth certificate and Byrne is campaigning for the British state to do something similar for donor-conceived children, by releasing the identity of their donors on request.

I understand the frustration, while also feeling sympathetic to donors who were promised their donation was a transitory and untraceable good deed. As it stands, donors can choose to withdraw their anonymity voluntarily, but very few have done so. I am lucky to know who my donor is.

Though in an age of online DNA tests, we must acknowledge that anonymity is a finite and fast-diminishing resource. It may not be long before Hettie can connect the dots herself, whether the donor is open to it or not.

A few months after her unsuccessful embryo transfer, Ella tried again with one of her six frozen embryos. A week before her thirty-eighth birthday, she sent me a photo of a positive pregnancy test. One of us had finally done it. I was thrilled for her.

Then I pictured us on our regular morning walks in the park, her pushing a pram and me walking alongside, alone. I had hoped that it would happen around the same time for us. Maybe next month I'll be pregnant too, I hoped. I wasn't single any more, and we were trying.

Art

Definition

1. The expression of human creativity and imagination
2. Paintings, drawings and sculptures
3. Assisted reproductive technology

Early on a July morning in 2024, I met Libby, my half-sister, at Gatwick Airport. Two weeks earlier Eliza, our Russian half-sister, had messaged our sibling WhatsApp group – named 'Need a kidney? No problem' – asking if any of us wanted to meet in Paris while she and her boyfriend were on holiday there. The Western sanctions against Russia since the Ukraine war had made it difficult for Russian citizens to get a visa for the UK, so it felt like a rare opportunity to meet her in person. Within days Libby and I had booked an impromptu trip to the French capital. In the years since we first met I had hung out with Libby and Lucy a couple of times a year and gotten to know them quite well. It would be fun to meet another half-sister.

After navigating ourselves from the airport to our hotel, we arranged to meet Eliza and her boyfriend, Nikita, at a typical French corner café, with woven chairs and metal tables perched on the pavement. I felt excited and a little jittery. Would there be any awkwardness? I wondered. Would our differences in culture and language keep us from connecting on anything but a surface level? We were sipping strong coffee when we spotted them walking over. We jumped up and hugged them. Eliza was shorter than I had pictured. Her smile was wide and striking, her skin dewy and radiant. Immediately the three of us started comparing ourselves while laughing, asking Nikita if he could see any resemblance between us.

As we walked towards the centre of Paris, my apprehensions evaporated; Eliza and Nikita were warm and easy to talk to. We paced the city streets like we were in a Richard Linklater film, walking and deep-talking like old friends who hadn't seen each other in years. Surprisingly, it didn't feel like there was much cultural difference at all. Like us, Eliza had grown up watching *Friends*, *Sex and the City* and *Girls*. She was a newly qualified psychologist and I enjoyed the nuance and expansiveness of our conversations. Within a few hours we were talking about nationality as a construct, the way power changes people and the work of psychologists in helping people to reshape their own narratives. I always thought that if I hadn't worked in television, I would have trained as a psychologist. Out of all the half-siblings – despite growing up a thousand miles apart – I felt most similar to Eliza.

Our first port of call was the Musée National d'Art Moderne at the Centre Pompidou. I had never been but always wanted to go. The building itself is something to behold. At first it appears to be plastered in scaffolding, obscuring the main event, then you realise, *Non!* It is meant to look like that, as if fashioned after a metal hamster cage, with human-sized tunnels and a giant red slide bolted on to the front. *L'art, je suppose.*

On the escalator up to the galleries, Libby noticed something.

'Wow, you guys both have similar tattoos on your arms,' she said.

I looked down and saw Eliza's tattoo: a small circle inside a larger one; a sun and moon conjoined. Simple thin black lines, just like mine.

'What are the chances?' I said, showing her the small sun and moon etched above my elbows.

'That's crazy,' Eliza said, smiling.

The three of us wandered around whispering and giggling and pointing at paintings, like children on a school trip. We took a selfie with Sylvia von Harden, depicted in her black and red plaid dress, copying her gormless expression and pretending to hold fake cigarettes between our fingers. We took a photograph of us reflected in a mirror of monochrome bleu. International Klein Blue. The most brilliant blue you'll ever see. 'Blue has no dimension,' Klein said, 'it is beyond dimensions.'

While we were roaming around the fifth floor, out of the corner of my eye I noticed her. All bright colours and eyebrow. Unmistakable. A small self-portrait of Frida Kahlo. I was shocked that I had never seen it before. *The Frame*, 1938. I didn't even know it existed. I kept rereading the plaque to check that it was definitely a self-portrait. It was, but the frame, painted with birds and flowers, had been made by Mexican craftspeople and bought by Kahlo from a market in Oaxaca. A frame within a frame.

I called Libby and Eliza over and we spent a while admiring the piece together.

When Kahlo exhibited her work in Paris in 1939, she was showered with praise by Picasso, Kandinsky and Tanguy on the opening night. Joan Miró even gave her a big hug. But of the eighteen paintings on offer, only *The Frame* found a buyer. It was the first time a female artist had ever sold a painting to the Louvre.

The Frame was painted not long after Kahlo met Leon Trotsky, the Soviet revolutionary. Kahlo and her husband, Diego Rivera, had been following the Russian revolution and the rise of Communism closely and considered Trotsky a hero. When the revolutionary was exiled from the USSR by Stalin, Rivera convinced the president of Mexico to grant him political asylum.

Russian Trotsky and Mexican Kahlo spoke in English – a language Trotsky's wife could not understand – and famously had a brief affair. It was a blow for Rivera, not only to be cheated on but with a man he admired so much and for whom he had called in a political favour. For Kahlo it was delicious revenge for the years of infidelity she had endured from her husband.

I dragged myself away from the self-portrait and continued wandering around the gallery on a high. A few hours later, the four of us left the Centre Pompidou and walked into a nearby deli.

'Libby, did we tell you about the letter from the Queen?' I said.

'What, no?' she replied.

I pulled out my phone and searched through my inbox. Four months earlier I had received an email from Simon Fishel, with two attachments. I opened the first and showed it to Libby. It was a photograph of two women sitting on a sofa, smiling. The woman on the left had tied-back grey hair, wore a green dress and was holding a small baby. Next to her was a younger woman with mid-length brown hair, oversized glasses, blue jeans and a red T-shirt with the words 'Patriots Dry Rum' on the front. She was holding another baby, swaddled in layers with a pacifier in their mouth.

'That's my mum and my grandma,' Eliza said. 'And that's me and Mike when we were a few months old.'

'Oh my goodness,' said Libby. 'What a precious photo.'

'Simon sent it to the Queen,' I said.

'Wow.'

'And he got a reply.'

I opened the second attachment. It was a scanned copy of a letter with the words 'Buckingham Palace' stamped at the top, dated 24 August 1993.

> The Queen was pleased to hear that you had been successful in helping Mrs. Popova and can understand how delighted she must be with healthy twins. Her Majesty thought it was kind of you to send the letter and I am to thank you for writing.

'That's so amazing,' Libby said.

'Two tiny newborns, bridging the gap between East and West,' I said.

'Well, we were named after Queen Elizabeth and Mikhail Gorbachev.'

'Oh my god,' Libby said, 'Eliza and Mike . . . I didn't realise!'

Libby and Lucy were born in 1990, the year the Berlin Wall was officially dismantled. I was born six months later, once the Soviet Union had formally collapsed. By 1993, Eliza, Mike and modern-day Russia had been born. But before the Iron Curtain fell, the USSR had not permitted its citizens to travel to the West.

Of the thousands of patients Simon Fishel had seen throughout his career, he remembered Eliza's mother clearly. She had appeared in his office one day asking for help, but being a student, she could not afford fertility treatment. Simon persuaded a drug company to supply the medication free of charge and offered her a significant discount. Ten months later he received a letter from her after she had moved back to St Petersburg.

Dear Dr Fishel,

You will be glad to learn that your IVF treatment of me in September 1992 turned out to be very successful and on May 14, 1993 I gave birth to twins – a boy and a girl.

The girl is very active and more a western smiling type. The boy likes to meditate and is more of a Russian thoughtful character.

We called the babies Michael and Elisabeth to remind us of our state leaders Mikhail Gorbachev and your queen Elizabeth II. In a way it was due to them that I had the chance to visit England and be treated in your clinic. I am grateful to you and Dr. Faratian personally for your great art – that is how I like to call it.

A few months before we met in Paris, Eliza and her mother had dug up the letter and sent it to me. I had wanted to find out more about Eliza's story so asked if we could chat over video call. She agreed happily, saying she had been doing some excavations into her family history herself.

'There's this word in Russian, Мутки,' Eliza said. 'It's pronounced "mootki". It comes from the word for "mud" or "swamp", specifically the bottom part where you can't see anything. Where everything is blurry, dirty and covered in darkness. That's the word my brother used.'

Eliza was talking about the moment she discovered how she was conceived.

'Metaphorically, we use the term to describe some shady business between two people that they don't open up about.'

When Eliza and Mike turned eighteen, their mother insisted on taking them on a trip to the UK, but that summer Eliza had planned to go on holiday to Italy with her friends instead, so her mum and brother flew to England without her. When they returned, her mum asked Eliza whether Mike had mentioned anything about the trip. Not really, she said, apart from that cryptic word: Мутки.

'So I said to Mum, "Can you please tell me what's going on?" And she just said, "Well, your dad is not your dad. I had IVF in England in 1992." And that was it. She just dropped it.

'So this is your dad that you've grown up with thinking is your dad your whole life,' Eliza continued, 'but I think my brother and I both kind of knew there was something weird because my mum gave birth to us when she was thirty-nine, and our dad, at the time, was almost sixty; twenty years older than her.'

In the early 1990s, when Eliza's mother was at university in St Petersburg, the sanctions between the East and West were dropped and citizens of the newly formed Russian Federation were finally allowed to travel more freely. Eliza's mother won a scholarship to study abroad and became one of the first students from modern Russia to do so in the West. She started a postgraduate degree in English at the University of Nottingham, where Simon Fishel was working, having set up a new fertility clinic and begun teaching the world's first Master's degree in ART: Assisted Reproductive Technology.

'I'm so grateful to her,' Eliza said. 'I think it's super brave to go and study abroad. She went to the UK to get her Master's degree when she was thirty-seven. She didn't know what she was doing, but she was paving the way for me to have my own freedom and kind of looking at the world and the narratives that surround women.'

Thirty-five years earlier, in the 1950s, scientists at the Crimean Medical Institute had been researching the artificial fertilisation of human eggs. In 1955 a postgraduate student reportedly transferred the embryo of an infertile couple – fertilised outside the body – into the woman's womb and she became pregnant. But thirteen weeks later she miscarried. If the reports are true, it means that the Soviet Union was decades ahead of the rest of the world with IVF. But when the Communist Party of the Soviet Union found out, they quickly banned the research, prohibiting 'experiments on Soviet women'.

When the first Russian IVF baby was eventually born in 1986, treatment was so expensive and inaccessible the children were nicknamed 'diamond babies'. As in the UK, the technology sparked immense criticism, particularly from religious groups, never mind the additional stigma of using donor sperm from a foreign country.

'Back then the Soviet Union was a closed country,' Eliza said, 'and the way it was governed had a big imprint on people's psychological states.' For many people, speaking up freely and talking about these kinds of things was scary. Eliza's mum never told anyone, aside from one of her best friends, and when she told her children, she asked them to keep it a secret. 'When there is a secret, there's a lot of shame around it,' said Eliza.

Knowing of her background in psychology, I was particularly intrigued by Eliza's thoughts about this kind of shame.

'How did you feel about her asking you to keep the secret?'

'I think I had anger at her, but at that point I also knew where it came from. She was born in 1954, the year after Stalin died, and she was always concerned about her privacy. She's concerned with who I've told about it, but by now I've told many of my friends, because, well, I think it's something about me now and it's not hers, so I think I have the right to do whatever I want with this information because it's about how I was conceived.'

I told Eliza it's something I think about a lot. Who do these stories belong to? Where do our stories start and our parents' stories end?

I asked about her dad.

'He was like the British monarch, a figurehead, with very little power,' she said. 'He was quite dark and anxious about things and not very present, so it was difficult to identify with him. I would say we had a distant relationship; we were never close. He died a few years ago, he was eighty-seven.' She never discussed the donor conception with him.

The idea to look for her donor came from her mother. Eliza's brother has suffered health issues for most of his life, but a few years ago doctors found a non-cancerous tumour in his brain. 'It's a pituitary gland tumour that produces prolactin,' she said, 'and my mum wanted to see if it was something genetic, so she and Mike wrote to the clinic.'

Since Eliza and Mike had been born in 1993, it meant they could go down the official route of HFEA records. Since 'Rodney', the donor, had voluntarily given up his right to anonymity, they were put in touch and in 2019, Eliza's brother and mother exchanged some emails with him. They kept Eliza updated, but she wasn't very interested. It is only in recent years, since training as a psychologist, that she has delved into her family's health and history and wanted to find out more.

I asked how it had felt being in touch with him.

'I don't think of him as my father or anything. He's smart and he's a scientist and he has a weird sense of humour. These kinds of things, I guess, let me know more about myself that I wasn't able to when looking at my dad. There's plenty of people who were donor-conceived who will never find out where they came from, so it's good to know something about him.'

Since the war with Ukraine has made travel difficult for Russians, now that Eliza has connected with Rodney she has toyed with the idea of trying to obtain a British passport through him. She spoke to a lawyer, who said it was unprecedented territory but worth a try.

'I'm not exactly Russian,' she said, 'but I'm not exactly *not* Russian. When I studied in the United States when I was sixteen, it left this big impression on me.'

Like her mother two decades before, Eliza won a scholarship to study abroad, part of an American exchange programme for post-Soviet countries funded by the Department of State. She was placed with a host family in Kansas City and lived with them for ten months.

Strangely enough, the American couple had been trying to conceive but didn't have any luck. They had tried IVF, but it didn't work and they ended up adopting three children from Russia.

'The three kids were natural siblings and they were from the same part of southern Russia that my grandfather is from,' said Eliza.

Fifteen years later, Eliza still keeps in touch with her host parents and has visited them since.

Before we ended the call, she mentioned a film that her dad used to watch while she was growing up. It was called Ширли-мырли or *What a Mess!*

'It was his favourite movie,' she said. 'It's a comedy about quadruplet siblings who were separated at birth and they find each other as adults. One of them is raised Jewish, another is raised Romani, another is raised Russian and the final one is raised in Africa. And they all hate each other, but then they kind of become friends. And so I'm thinking like, was there something that my dad was trying to tell us?'

I wondered if it was her dad's way of making peace with how Eliza and her brother were conceived.

'I think we're in this weird place in the progress of the world and how it's developing,' she said. 'And soon it will be just a normal thing that, you know, we're born from everywhere and it's a beautiful thing, really, because it does break down those barriers of hatred.'

I asked Eliza to send me a link to the film so I could watch it. It begins with the discovery of an enormous diamond in the Russian Far East. They call it the 'Saviour of Russia' and the government announces a plan to use it to pay off all of Russia's national debt. When the film was released in 1995, as the newly formed Russian Federation headed towards a financial crisis, it was the kind of miracle they could only dream of. Meanwhile, for those who dream of their own little miracles, ART has become a routine part of medical treatment in Russia today, even being state-funded as part of the government's plan to boost birth rates. Diamonds, it seems, have become much more affordable.

In Paris it was warm but windy and overcast. We walked along the Seine and stopped to take photos when we reached the Eiffel Tower. Five colourful circles stood out against the grey. It was two weeks before the Olympic Games were due to start and there was a glut of activity along the river; viewing platforms being constructed and temporary structures draped in the pink and purple banners of 'Paris 2024'.

Because of the war in Ukraine, Russian athletes were banned from competing, aside from a few who had been approved to compete as 'Individual Neutral Athletes'.

'What do British people think of Russians?' Eliza asked.

I paused and thought carefully about my words.

'I guess I associate Russia with great literature, classical music, ballet dancers and models,' I said. 'But obviously, we don't like the war.'

'You see my cardigan and bag?' she said.

'Yeah,' I replied, looking at her yellow cardigan and baby blue bag.

'I would have to be careful wearing this in Russia. There may be no KGB any more, but there are still people watching. The other week we were going to walk through one of the main squares in St Petersburg and Nikita noticed I was wearing these at the same time, so I changed bags.'

'Oh, gosh,' I said. 'I didn't realise it was that bad.'

'You are a nobody in Russia until you speak out loud about politics. Then, in the government's eyes, you become a very important person.'

We got the Metro back to our hotel and a few hours later Eliza arrived in the lobby and presented us with a gift bag each. On the front of the bag was Great Gostiny Dvor, a grand building in St Petersburg and one of the oldest shopping malls in the world. Inside was a silk scarf, a gold-plated porcelain mug and a bag of wafer chocolates, all traditional and handmade. I was touched that Eliza had brought us such beautiful gifts all that way; it was so unexpected and kind. From Russia with love.

That night we went to the Moulin Rouge, ordered champagne and enjoyed one of the most entertaining evenings of my life. Everything was so decadent, so velvet, so sparkling, so red and so nude. We sat in the front row and while the others faced the stage, my seat was virtually on top of it. Whenever a dancer with a particularly flamboyant outfit walked past I got a face full of feathers, causing Libby and Eliza to cackle in hysterics.

We shared our photos on Instagram and tagged each other: '36 heures à Paris avec les demi sœurs,' I wrote in the caption. It was the first time I had shared anything publicly about my half-siblings. I was no longer keeping the secret from anyone and when I uploaded the post I felt a little lighter.

I tagged Eliza, then clicked on her profile and noticed a sentence written in Russian on her bio.

наши пути здесь, конечно, имеют грани подобия, потому что все едино

I copied and pasted it into Google Translate.

Our paths here, of course, have edges of similarity, because everything is one.

Half

Definition

1. Two equal parts
2. One of a pair
3. Falling short of a complete thing

'I like to wind people up a bit,' Hettie told me. 'I tell people I'm half-Polish, half-Scottish, and they're like, oh, on which side? And I say, well, I've never met my dad. And they usually say something like, "Oh, so they broke up before you were born?" And I say, "No, my mum's never met him either."' She paused. 'And then I just wait for their reaction.'

I wanted to speak to Dorothy Byrne's daughter, Hettie, to find out more about life as a donor-conceived child from a single parent family. Hettie, now in her late twenties, also works in television production and we had arranged to chat over video call during her lunch break one Friday afternoon.

'I suppose it's nice to think that I was really wanted, and I wasn't, you know, just a kid that was born because something happened between two people.'

'Do you want to know more about your donor?' I asked.

'I don't think I've missed out on anything, it would just be nice to know why he did it. Because part of me thinks, oh he probably just did it for the money. Like in *Friends*, Joey just does it because he's broke. Or was he doing it because he had kids already and thought, oh my God my kids are so great, I want to pass on my genetics? You just have no idea. So it's a kind of curiosity really.'

Hettie has a young face and a brown bob with a middle parting. She wore a velvet, sleeveless turtleneck top, reminiscent of the nineties fashion from the time she was born.

I asked if she had made peace with the idea that she might never know any more about the donor.

'It would be hard to let me down because I have no expectations. I don't really think about it because I've always known. I think it would be cool to know more, but I probably won't and I'll just keep going on with my life like I have been.'

'There's a difference between desperation and just normal curiosity isn't there,' I said. 'You don't feel like you're missing a big piece of your life, like people expect you to.'

'Exactly, although I do wonder about when I hopefully have children, especially if they look a bit different to my family, maybe then I'll have a bit more of a sense of longing compared to a sense of curiosity.'

Hettie was relaxed and easygoing when we talked. For me, discussing such topics has always been wrapped up in secrecy and angst, so it was refreshing to speak to someone so calm and assured in their feelings about it. Aside from my siblings, she is the only person I've talked to with first-hand experience of being donor-conceived.

'I've always thought,' Hettie said, 'and especially talking to you, that I'd like being able to talk to someone who knows exactly what's going on, who has all the information, where you don't have to start from zero in explaining your whole life and what all these little acronyms are, or how the law is different now.' I nodded in agreement. 'So I think in that way, I'd like to know my siblings just to have that sort of kinship. And then if we all had kids, seeing how they look in comparison to us.'

The HFEA informed Hettie that she has at least eight

half-siblings. She signed up to some DNA websites and two half-siblings have come up, but one's profile is private and the other has not replied to her message. If any of them were born after 2005 when the anonymity law changed, there is more hope of finding out, through them, who her donor is, but it would mean a substantial age gap of eight years or more between siblings.

Hettie asked about my half-siblings and I explained the different ways we'd discovered we were donor-conceived, including my family's secret.

'Do you think there's ever a benefit to keeping it a secret?' I asked her.

'No. I understand the whole sensitivity of it if they have two parents, but then it's who you are, it's what you look like, it's the sicknesses you might get, it's how young you'll be when your hair goes grey. Do you have certain passions or issues that can't be explained from your parents? You have to do it in a way that's sensitive and respectful of how your child might react. I mean, you just have to do it all from love. But yeah, times have changed so much, I just don't think it should be kept from anyone these days, I feel quite passionately about that.'

'And for parents who are worried or insecure that their child might, you know, find this other family, what would you say to them?'

'I mean, there are a lot of reasons that your kids could hate you. It probably won't be that one.'

I laughed. It was a really good answer.

For Hettie, and many other donor-conceived children, half of her medical history remains blank.

'When I was younger,' she said, 'I had to have an operation on my legs for a hereditary, genetic condition, and it's not from my mum's side of the family. So I was like, the bastard gave me a reason to have an operation for goodness' sake.'

Like her mum, Hettie is effortlessly funny.
'He also gave me life, but I suppose no one's perfect.'

In the years since I told my siblings the truth, my older brother, Tim, decided to sign up to a DNA website too. He was matched with a half-brother, two years younger than him. Tim sent a message and the man replied asking if he knew anything about the scenario of his conception. Yes, Tim said: IVF with a male donor. The half-brother responded saying he was glad Tim was aware, it could have been a 'very eye opening conversation otherwise!'

Tim sent me a link to his Facebook profile.

> He doesn't look much like you

>> Haha yeah he doesn't, guess that's the wonder of genetics and everyone carrying two different versions of everything within them.

A few months later, my own half-siblings arranged a meet-up in London. Since the Christmas revelation, I have regularly checked in with Ruth and Joe about how they feel and whether they want any more information about the donor or siblings. Neither showed much interest until recently, two years after finding out, so I invited them to the gathering. Ruth was on a cruise ship for a whale survey around the Canary Islands so she joined by video call, along with Eliza in Russia.

When Joe and I arrived at the bar in south London, Ben, Libby and Lucy were already there. It was a 'doodle bar' with black chalkboards surrounding our table. I burst out laughing when I saw that Libby, a professional artist and signmaker, had written 'Sperm Donor Kids' in huge bubble letters on the wall, complete with giant sperm and Rodney's favourite specialist subjects: ants and mushrooms. We asked someone on the next table to take a photo of us all in front of it, and I held up my phone so that Ruth and Eliza's tiny faces – livestreamed from different continents – were included too.

We had a fun night – underpinned by our mutual dark sense of humour – enjoying a meal at a Mexican restaurant and then a pub before we hugged, said our goodbyes and set off in different directions. The next day Ben changed our group chat name to 'Tossed Together'.

I had felt so alone when my parents reluctantly admitted how we were conceived and we agreed to keep it a secret. I had no idea that years down the line I would be laughing and joking with other people who knew exactly what it felt like, including my own triplet siblings.

'Humour cuts through shame,' Rodney had said on our video call, and I couldn't agree more.

Crazy

Definition

1. Mentally ill
2. Extremely enthusiastic
3. Stupid or unreasonable

Last night I dreamed I was having a miscarriage. Among the blood was a small spine, the size and shape of a fish bone. I think it *was* a fish bone. Other times I dream that I am pregnant or nursing.

A few weeks ago I received the results back from another fertility blood test. One hormone came back abnormally high. Prolactin. Its main function is to produce milk for breastfeeding. Was I having a phantom pregnancy? Were my dreams telling my body that I really wanted a baby? Unfortunately, having a high amount of this hormone when you're not pregnant is bad for fertility. Another way my body was fighting against me. I waited six weeks to have my blood retested to find out which of three possibilities was causing the abnormal result: a random anomalous spike, a sign of stress or a symptom of a pituitary gland brain tumour, like Mike, my half-brother.

When I was a child, we had a dog called Pepsi who had a phantom pregnancy. She lactated milk from her teats and gathered all her soft toys and our slippers into her bed, as if they were puppies. I felt sorry for her and tried to help when she got distressed looking for one of her 'puppies'. In humans, this phenomenon is called pseudocyesis or 'false pregnancy'. In the past it was referred to as 'hysterical' or 'delusional' pregnancy.

Historians have noted a string of pseudocyesis in British queens, including Anne Boleyn, Mary I of England and Queen Anne. This does not surprise me. The psychological pressure of producing an heir to the throne must have been immense for a monarch. For some, their life literally depended on it. After she suffered two miscarriages and a stillbirth, Henry VIII ordered his second wife, Anne Boleyn, to be beheaded. She had given him a daughter, but he wanted a son.

Henry VIII had six wives and of their combined pregnancies 70 per cent ended in miscarriage or stillbirth. His wives were blamed – and consequently divorced and murdered – but it's quite likely the issue lay with him. Of the two sons who did survive infancy (though not to adulthood), one was illegitimate (conceived with a maid) and therefore not eligible as an heir, and the other was born to Henry's 'favourite wife', Jane Seymour, who died from complications of childbirth. After watching her father execute her mother when she was two years old, Henry's daughter, Elizabeth I, chose a life of celibacy, free from the pressures of marriage and procreation.

I spoke to a TV friend recently who for years struggled to conceive and, like me, had done all the research about improving her chances. On the list of things to be avoided were plastic containers because they can leach toxins into food and drinks. But on a hot summer's day at work, she realised she had forgotten her steel water bottle. Anxious about her fertility, she didn't want to drink from the free plastic water bottles provided at the office, so, paralysed with indecision, she ended up stressed and dehydrated. Being faced with so much uncertainty about what is causing us not to conceive can drive us crazy. It was a turning point, she said.

She also told me how she'd become envious of other people's

miscarriages, which I can relate to. At least their bodies can do something, I think, then berate myself. And there is also the envy of other people's reactions. The grief around miscarriage is legitimate and acknowledged. We gather around in support, offering love and kind words, but no one does that when you have a period, crushed by the wrecking ball of infertility every month. No one gathers round when your partner tells you he is not ready, while endometriosis eats away at your eggs. Or when you don't have a partner.

If I sound bitter, it's because I am. And I go on hating myself for thinking these things.

Soon after I started my IVF medication, I sat on the sofa shuffling a deck of tarot cards. Very aware that I was like a mad woman trying to predict the future, I asked the spirits, or whoever, what the outcome of the IVF would be. Out came the 'three of swords', my least favourite card. The image showed a big red heart being tugged in different directions, ripping at the seams. Below it a young woman, eyes closed, screaming into the sky. The background was grey and desolate, aside from a single skeletal tree. I was so alarmed that I called James over. I told him I was worried it might mean a negative pregnancy test or a miscarriage. I had no idea that a totally different devastating outcome was even possible.

'Heartbroken, she falls to her knees, and screams to the Universe for a second chance,' the card read. 'What happened? Why did she have this taken from her?'

I was too demanding, too unlovable, I wanted too much. I broke my own heart.

Some couples stay together for the kids and some break up to avoid having them. In the months since James left I have reflected on what the years of waiting and wanting have done to me and the people I love. Infertility was holding me hostage, causing me to act out then apologise, self-sabotage then desperately circle back. Like Miss Havisham, I remain in my wedding dress with the clocks stopped, mourning something I haven't lost yet. But in the meantime I'm losing myself.

In 2012, three gynecological surgeons, the Nezhat brothers, published a groundbreaking paper solving 'a centuries old mystery'. For hundreds of years women had been diagnosed with something called 'hysteria' and cruelly subjected to 'murder, madhouses, and lives of unremitting physical, social, and psychological pain'. But, 'in the majority of cases' they claimed, most were likely suffering with endometriosis.

The ancient Greeks believed uterine distress of young widows to be 'a result of their loss of sexual fulfilment' and to have driven them to 'madness'. By the eighteenth century, an entirely opposite theory had been proposed: females liable to nymphomania, promiscuity or depravity caused pelvic pain and hysteria. Women must have enough sexual desire, but not too much. 'Faced with such injustices,' the researchers wrote, 'women with endometriosis have been contemplating or committing suicide for centuries.'

Victorian gynaecologist Dr Isaac Baker Brown reported that 'in almost all hysterical patients' there was an 'exacerbation at the menstrual periods'. As he was a fellow of the Royal College of Surgeons and one of the founders of St Mary's Hospital in London, where he was chief obstetrician, you might count yourself lucky to be in the hands of such an accomplished doctor. But in his 1866 published medical paper, Baker Brown conflated low libido, miscarriage and infertility with madness. 'A distaste for marital intercourse, and very frequently either sterility or a tendency to abort in the early months of pregnancy,' he wrote, 'these physical evidences of derangement, if left unchecked, gradually lead to more serious consequences. The patient either becomes a confirmed invalid, always ailing, and confined to bed or sofa, or on the other hand, will become subject to catalepsy, epilepsy, idiotcy, or insanity.'

His cure for such 'nervous diseases' was to perform a type of surgery called a clitoridectomy. 'Having been placed completely under the influence of chloroform,' he explained, 'the clitoris is freely excised either by scissors or knife – I always prefer the scissors.' At least forty-eight girls and women were subjected to Baker Brown's scissors before he was eventually expelled from the Obstetrical Society of London for performing the operations without their consent.

Infertility is like acne. Everyone with naturally flawless skin likes to give you advice. Have you tried washing your face with soap or drinking more water? Have you tried tea tree oil or being less stressed? My sister's best friend swears by X or Y or Z. But the fact is, you just have different skin; your hormones and biology are different. Improving your lifestyle generally – getting more sleep, keeping hydrated, eating less junk – might help, but it probably isn't the difference between those who have acne and those who don't. Being fit and healthy does not protect you from infertility or the natural ageing of your ovarian supply. Some young, fit and healthy women will have a poor egg reserve and some older, unhealthy women will have a good egg reserve. As one of the most health-conscious among my friends, it is frustrating to accept this. When I filmed the midwife television series I watched pregnant women smoking outside the hospital doors. In other jobs I have come across heavy drinkers, career criminals and people living the most turbulent lifestyles with five or six children. In the street I sometimes see obese parents and their obese children eating junk food and I wonder how our bodies can function so differently. I feel bad for judging, I try not to. I'm just sad.

The writer Haley Nahman has described the 'cognitive dissonance of trying to conceive'. Against your better judgement infertility can start to take over your every waking thought, and you begin to resent it. It starts to pervade almost everything you do, everywhere you go. When I leave the house I see pregnant bellies and prams everywhere. When I go to the gym or supermarket, the car park separates the 'parents and children' from everyone else. Each time I watch television I am asked if I want to 'add child' or 'adjust parental controls'. Every time I log on to social media I am pulled into a torrent of birth announcements, baby showers, birthday parties and wholesome family photos. I am bombarded by adverts for fertility tests warning me not to leave it too late and suggested posts to clear my chakras or buy supplements that will help me 'get pregnant within three cycles'. I change my settings, but the gullet punches keep on coming.

I know that men are not subject to such a skirmish by their algorithms. There are no adverts from semen analysis companies scaremongering men into parting with their cash 'before it's too late'.

I have a subscription for expensive crushed seeds because of a podcast that claimed 'seed cycling' can help you get pregnant. I recently bought cough syrup to drink around ovulation because of a TikTok trend that said it loosens your cervical mucus. I have had my vagina and gut microbiomes tested in faraway labs, and then taken pre- and probiotics to try and improve them. Aside from the financial cost, researching and ordering these things have taken up so much of my time.

There is a point when hoping starts to hurt. When the desire has gone for so long unattended, the prayers for so long unanswered, that the wanting caves in on itself. I know it would be much easier to *not* want to be a mother, and sometimes I wonder if I really do. I see my friends with kids having their own problems. I am unable to hold a conversation with them for more than thirty seconds without a child interrupting or crying. I picture a life of demanding toddlers, snotty noses and weekends spent at sticky soft play. Why would I want that? Why am I so eager to give up my freedom?

Then I remember the man I filmed on a psychedelic retreat years ago, besotted with and humbled by his newborn twins.

'I thought, as their father, it was going to be me teaching them things,' he said, 'but I'm the one who has been learning from them.'

And I think of my friend, Ally, who writes the most beautiful words on Instagram about life as a mother.

> I used to kind of roll my eyes whenever I'd read a caption like, 'being your mom is the greatest thing in the world!' but the joke's on me with that one.
>
> For all the dramatics surrounding your arrival, a sweet layer of serenity has washed over our lives since you came. I love who you've made me and who I've become as a result of you, your need and your love. Thank you for making me a person that I love, too. It's true what they say, that maternity is a pairing of bliss and survival.

Bliss and survival.

All I know is that I want a family like the one I have. I want a busy house of people talking over each other at the dinner table and Easter egg hunts and Christmas gingerbread house building competitions. I want all that love and chaos.

There are few things in life you have to commit to blindly. No one knows what being a parent will be like, but by the time they've done it, it's too late to turn back. As I've stepped into my thirties I have also battled with how wanting to be a mother fits in with my feminist values.

'The option to decide whether we want to have kids, and who we want to have kids with,' wrote Ruby Warrington in her book *Women Without Kids*, 'is a privilege that has been won by decades – if not centuries – of feminist resistance, and the fight for gender equality.'

Sometimes I feel bad for wanting something that women have fought to have the option to avoid. I read accounts of older women who have aged into poverty because – after being widowed or divorced – they are paid less in their jobs, having had to drop in and out of the workforce to look after their children, and often their elderly parents too. They have missed years of opportunities at work that their partners have not. In financial terms, having children affects women far more disproportionately than men. There is still so much inequality in child-rearing.

Despite all the ways my mum has broken free of the expectations for women of her time – travelling the world, running her own business, undergoing fertility treatment – she does not describe herself as a feminist. In her experience, the Second Wave Feminism movement, which began when she was in her teens, seemed to pile on more problems rather than taking them away. As a young woman I confidently rebutted this. Of course the liberation of women has been a positive thing, I would say, it gives us the *choice*.

I messaged her to see if her opinion had changed in recent years.

> Would you describe yourself as a feminist?

> **No**

> Because it meant that women were expected to do it all – work AND look after children?

> **You could choose to be just a housewife**

> **Men used to earn enough on their own to support their families**

> You could still choose that now?

> Not really because most households now need two incomes
>
> I didn't need to be a feminist to choose to work
>
> Even though feminism means equality?
>
> I've never seen it that way
>
> But that's literally what it means
>
> Each partner in a relationship does what they are best at.
>
> That's why I'm not a feminist.
>
> I don't want to be equal. I want to choose.

While I'm not entirely sure what she means, I do not press her further. My mother's relationship with feminism no longer frustrates me like it used to. I feel deep compassion for a woman who had to study and work while raising four children, at the same time as looking after her elderly mother and uncle. Alongside the menopause and driving us to sports and drama clubs and dentist appointments and friends' houses. Doing the food shop and cooking for six people every day. Cleaning the house, doing the laundry, feeding the pets. Writing special notes from the tooth fairy, staying up all night on Christmas Eve to wrap mountains of presents and cheering us on at every swimming gala. Helping us with homework and planning birthdays and holidays and keeping track of everything and everyone. These were all my mum's jobs. There was little room for anything else, never mind having a social life. Once, she forgot to go to her own birthday party. Her friends waited for hours at the restaurant before realising she wasn't coming.

I was listening to a podcast recently in which Anna Whitehouse, founder of Mother Pukka and campaigner for flexible-working for parents, repeated something her therapist had said:

'Women are so angry right now, an anger that I have not seen, ever. They are angry at a world that raised them to think they could have it all and actually they've ended up doing it all.'

On an Instagram post she elaborated:

This is a generation of mothers trying to hold down a career under the weight of domestic / mental load and we're, frankly, exhausted. Exhausted of trying to explain it even. Exhausted of thinking non-stop about what everyone needs and losing ourselves among it all. And hacked off with employers not giving a hint of flexibility. Oh and making us redundant at one of the most vulnerable times in a woman's life. So yeah, almost too tired to be angry. The maternal burnout is real.

Life as a woman can feel concertinaed. You have fifteen years to finish your education, flourish in your career, find your forever partner, get married, buy a house and have babies. But all the while you must have fun and not take life too seriously. That's the most common desire from men on dating apps.

Wants someone who . . . doesn't take themselves too seriously.

You must work hard (or inherit enough) to have chunks of savings left over for hobbies, holidays and other people's hen parties, baby showers and weddings. By the time you've done all this you might be thirty-five or so, also known as 'advanced maternal age' or a 'geriatric mother'. By then you might be too old to have more than one child. For some it might be too old to have even one. So, really, we're looking at somewhere in the five years between twenty-seven and thirty-two to have your first baby. Unless you want three children in total, in which case – according to mathematical research published in the *Human Reproduction* journal – you should start trying to conceive at age twenty-three. If you want two, you should start at age twenty-seven. By thirty-five, the odds are fifty-fifty. Every day I am drowning in numbers and statistics that seem only to be projectile-vomited at women. For many men – revelling in their extended adolescence – reproduction is something to be leaned into leisurely, in their mid-thirties at the very earliest. Like trying to feed a wild animal, you can't force it. Coax it gently, lest you scare it away. Reminders about ovulation windows are off-putting and any mention of sex for procreation is deeply unsexy. They would rather not engage in the calendar gymnastics and mental arithmetic that trying to conceive necessitates for their partner.

While we are told to start trying yesterday, men are told they can wait until tomorrow. I have met so many men who say they will probably start thinking about having kids when they hit forty, the age when most women are relieved that they can finally stop thinking about it.

I know several men who have left their wives and families to start a relationship with a much younger woman and had a second family in their fifties. With one, there is a twenty-seven-year age gap between children. Men seem to get a second shot if they want it, while women tend to get just one.

With globally declining birth rates, I've noticed certain news headlines becoming more common:

> Leaving It Too Late? Average Age of Starting IVF Passes 35
> Women are jeopardising their chance of having babies, regulator warns.

Almost every article about fertility refers exclusively to women, implying they are irresponsible for delaying motherhood and 'choosing' to have children later in life. There is not enough mention of the economical and societal factors causing the delay, or the non-age-related reasons for requiring fertility treatment. But most infuriatingly, there is a gaping absence of men. There seem to be a lot of 'childless women' but rarely any 'childless men'. It's as if all women are procreating entirely on their own.

Sperm quality has been declining dramatically for fifty years. Issues with sperm are responsible for a significant proportion of infertility. As men age, their sperm slows down. The risk of miscarriage increases when fathers pass forty and children born to older fathers are more likely to have autism, schizophrenia and leukaemia. First-time fathers are, on average, three years older than first-time mothers, but for some reason they are excluded from criticism by the media. It is women who are chastised because their ovaries do not produce babies immediately after having shut them off for a decade on the pill. Or because long waiting lists mean they are older than they wanted to be, or because they can't afford ten grand a go at IVF on top of a house deposit and mortgage. Not to mention the women like me who waited for their partner to be ready during their fertile years, only for them to change their mind at the final hurdle. Eight years of being told *not yet*.

In trying to hasten having children, I have probably, inadvertently, slowed it down. Any whiff of desperation is lethal, I discovered, even when communicated as a deep, human desire like any other. I took it all too seriously: my diagnosis, the doctor's advice, the double-speed clock. A year after I was abandoned, I am reminded over and over how important it is to do it with the right person. Though what, I can't help but wonder, if that is in lieu of doing it at all?

'It's a good job you didn't have a baby with him,' everyone tells me. But I notice that sentiment doesn't apply to couples who have children and then split up. Once a child exists there are different rules. No regrets, they are perfect. The ghost child, however, is wished away and forgotten, inconvenient and better off never living. Is it better not to have children at all than to have them with someone you won't stay with forever? In a world of separated and divorced parents, it would be a shame to think so.

When Marilyn Monroe was a child, her mother, Gladys, showed her a photo of a man and told her he was her father. It was a different man to the one whose name was written on her birth certificate, but knowing nothing about either man, Monroe was delighted.

'It felt so good to have a father,' she said, 'to be able to look at his picture and know I belonged to him.' He wore his hat to one side and had a thin moustache, and she thought he looked like the actor Clark Gable.

'I asked my mother what his name was. She wouldn't answer, but went into the bedroom and locked herself in.'

His name, Marilyn later discovered, was Stanley Charles Gifford and he was a co-worker of her mother's at a film company. They had been having an affair – he was married with children – and when Gladys told him she was pregnant he abandoned her. Not long after the conversation with her mother, Monroe started a scrapbook and the first picture she put in was a photograph of Clark Gable. Throughout her life, even at the height of her fame, Monroe tried to contact Gifford, but he always rebuffed her, leaving her deeply disappointed each time.

By 1960, now an icon herself, Monroe had made friends with her stand-in dad, Clark Gable, starring alongside him in a film called *The Misfits*.

'I'm sure he won't mind if I say it,' she said, 'because in a Freudian sense it's supposed to be very good – I used to always think of him as my father, I pretended that he was my father.' The film, written by Monroe's husband, Arthur Miller, was tipped to be a huge success. Monroe had even turned down the role of

Holly Golightly in *Breakfast at Tiffany's* to star in it. But the shoot, in the scorching Nevada desert, turned out to be difficult for many reasons, including coinciding with Monroe and Miller's divorce. Then, twelve days after filming ended, Gable suffered a heart attack and died.

Monroe was exhausted; grieving her marriage, her faux father and her real one. A week after *The Misfits* was released, she asked her psychoanalyst for help. She was admitted to a clinic, hoping for some rest and recuperation, but instead found herself locked in a padded room on a psychiatric ward.

'There was no empathy,' she wrote in a letter to her psychiatrist. 'It had a very bad effect – they asked me after putting me in a "cell" (I mean cement blocks and all) for <u>very disturbed</u> depressed patients except I felt I was in some kind of prison for a crime I hadn't committed. The inhumanity there I found archaic.' She went on to describe how the psychiatrist had performed a physical examination of her breasts for no reason, and being told by the man in charge that she was 'a very, very sick girl and had been a very, very sick girl for many years'.

The next day the *New York World-Telegram* reported that Monroe was 'undergoing treatment as a highly disturbed patient', having been 'frightened and desperately depressed by a life of shattered marriages and sordid childhood experiences'. This referred to the sexual abuse she had experienced from the age of eight by a man who rented a room from her foster parents. Marilyn was tormented from all angles, with no escape route. Not even the doctors would help her.

As she grew older, I think Monroe hoped that having a child might help to heal her own childhood wounds.

'It's one of the things I dream of,' she said. 'I know how I'll bring her up – without lies. Nobody will tell her lies about anything.'

Story

Definition

1. A narrative of real or imagined events
2. A report in a newspaper
3. A lie

When I was eleven, our class received a homework assignment to write a biography of one of our parents. Joe chose Dad, and Ruth and I chose Mum. Our parents told us stories we had never heard before – about emigrating to Australia, breeding dogs and travelling the world – and I was enthralled. I asked them questions, my first experience of interviewing. Mum dug up some old photographs from the attic and I included them in the homework – painstakingly scanning them into the computer and uploading them into a Word document – hoping I would get extra marks. Most of the pictures dated from my parents' time in Australia. In one Mum is wearing a crop top and shorts and holding two baby wallabies. In another she poses behind a massive palm tree leaf, her blonde hair and white shorts luminous in the sun. I had never seen her like this; wearing young person clothes. I had never seen them as people before they were parents. I had only seen Elvis, and that had been a mirage.

Two weeks later, I printed all seven pages, put them in a clear plastic sleeve and tied them together with small green treasury tags. I handed the homework to my teacher, beaming with pride.

By October 2023 I had finished my television contract and started a full-time Master's degree in creative writing at the University of Manchester. On my Monday morning commute from Leeds, my sat nav would sometimes take me through Oldham, and I would think about how fitting it was that I had ended up so close to the hospital where IVF was invented – while writing about my family's own story.

When James left I had to start paying full rent and bills on my own. As a full-time student, it was terrible timing. My savings would keep me going for a while, but I worried I would have to move back home.

Around this time, I received an email from Rodney. Among his usual hypotheses and links to scientific papers, he asked if I might help him write a 'manual' that would include not only his medical theories but the story of his life. He wanted me to be his ghostwriter.

'I am sure you might need the extra cash,' he wrote.

A sense of dread swelled in my body. I did need the money, more than ever, but I knew – immediately and deep within my bones – that it was something I could never agree to. Among the break-up and Sophie's diagnosis, the world had already stopped making sense. Ghostwriting for my own sperm donor seemed both perfectly logical and also completely insane. It was too meta, too much.

He said there was no pressure, but the suggestion itself threw me. I took a few weeks to respond.

'I'm afraid I'll have to pass,' I replied. 'The complications with my family (and all the emotion surrounding the donor-conception secret and my dad in particular) mean that I wouldn't feel comfortable taking on that kind of a role unfortunately.

'I'm also experiencing a very difficult period of my life at the moment,' I continued, briefly explaining what had happened with James. 'I could do with the money, but I think the heaviness of everything right now is too much already without taking anything else on.'

Rodney responded with a quote from *The Unbearable Lightness of Being* by Milan Kundera.

'The heavier the burden,' it began, 'the closer our lives come to the earth, the more real and truthful they become.'

It's a book I happen to love. I had been sitting on a plane next to Sam when I read it five years earlier. We were flying to Toronto to see his family. At one point I was so enchanted by the way Kundera expressed something – one of those turns of phrase that made me feel understood on a deeply human level – that I asked Sam if I could read it aloud to him. He said he wasn't in the right headspace to listen. We were on a long-haul flight, I said, surely now was as good a time as any?

'It would mean a lot to me and will only take, like, twenty seconds. I think it might help you understand me better.'

But he stood his ground. It wasn't a good time. And I knew it never would be; it never was. It was such a minor moment in our relationship, but so damaging. It felt like he was rejecting my soul, my essence, my love of words, everything I treasured. He didn't want to understand me better, even when I begged him to, even when we were suspended in the sky, waiting for the hours to pass.

The chasm between us expanded. I never shared the quote with him and he never asked me about it again. I buried it, but Rodney's email brought it back. Rodney valued these things too. He knew how literature and language can make us feel seen, and help us to heal. It was comforting that we had found meaning in the same book, even if we were not on the same page.

★

In terms of keeping myself afloat – financially and psychologically – I realised I needed to write down my own story and have a stab at getting it published. I had planned to pitch it to literary agents the following year, after gaining some insight from my writing course, but I didn't have time. The month I started my Master's, I finished my book proposal and sent it to a handful of literary agents. When most of them replied to me, some within just a day or two, I cried with relief. I realised that not only was my story worth telling but that I could possibly forge a career as a writer, something I had dreamed of as a child.

But there was one final hurdle. I needed my family's support. I couldn't publish a story about our lives without them being on board and, having guarded the secret for so many years, I had no idea how they would react.

A couple of weeks later I went home for Bonfire Night and approached Mum.

'Mum, can I talk to you on your own for a second?'

'Okay,' she said.

She followed me upstairs and we sat on the bathroom step with the door closed.

'I don't know if this will be a surprise to you or not, since I've started a degree in creative writing,' I said. 'But I've been writing about the family secret.'

'Right,' she said, eyes wide open; neither shocked nor expectant.

'At first I thought it might just make an interesting article, but then lots of things have happened over the last few years and I realised it's a bigger story. And you know I've always wanted to be a writer, so I thought I would see if anyone was interested.'

'Oh, okay.' She looked a little dazed.

'And it turns out that they are. I emailed some agents and lots got back to me . . . and I've met with some who have offered to represent me. But, obviously, before I go any further I wanted to check if you and Dad and everyone else is okay with that?' Mum looked ahead, deep in thought.

'I'm okay with it,' she said finally. 'I've actually thought about writing down my own stories over the years, you know, of having IVF and triplets and everything.'

'Oh,' I said, surprised and moved to hear this. 'Well, I'd love to hear more of your stories, maybe I can include them in the book.'

'By the way, I'm sorry,' she said. 'When it first came out, I was trying to protect Dad but I realise it was probably at the expense of you. We just wanted things to carry on as normal.'

'I know,' I said.

We agreed that I should speak to Dad next, then my siblings. We enjoyed our annual Bonfire Night festivities and after everyone else went home, Mum, Dad and I were left alone in the garden room, now finally finished. With its huge oak beams and cosy wraparound leather sofa, it had quickly become everyone's favourite room of the house. The stained-glass lead lights above us were dim and Dad looked like he was falling asleep.

'Dad, can I talk to you about something?' I said, quietly. The words felt sharp and familiar in my mouth. I really hoped it would be the last time I had to start a conversation like this.

'Yeah, what's up?'

'Well, you know how I'm doing a writing degree at the moment. Do you remember what you said when I first told you I wanted to do it?'

'No.'

'You said "Writers don't make any money."'

'Did I?' he laughed.

'Yeah. Well, I was worried about that too, but I applied for my course with a story in mind, hoping to publish it one day.'

'Right,' he said.

'And it turns out that there are people who are interested in publishing it.'

'Oh, that's good.'

'But the story is about our family. It's about IVF and infertility and me and my problems and yours and Mum's journey.' I breathed. 'But it's also about the sperm donor and the secret and stuff.'

Dad's eyes narrowed and he nodded slightly.

'So before I go any further with it, I want to check how you feel about that. Mum said she is okay with it, but obviously . . . if you'd rather I didn't then that's fine, I won't—'

'Becka,' he interrupted, then paused. 'I'm one hundred per cent behind you.'

I felt like I was floating out of my body.

'In fact, I reckon we should open a bottle of prosecco to celebrate.'

I had thought he would need some time to think about it. My parents are not open books, they are private people who live like hermits in a forest with a menagerie of pets and go days without speaking to anyone else. Four years earlier Dad had celebrated us *not* telling anyone about the secret and now he was celebrating my decision to tell the whole world. It was the opposite of shame.

'I don't want to be famous,' Dad said as we sipped sparkling wine from golden flutes.

'Don't worry about that,' I smiled. 'I'll make sure there's no paparazzi at the door.'

'I'm dead proud of you, darling,' he said.

Seven weeks later, the family was gathered again for Christmas. Throughout the games, meals and long walks, I spoke to Ruth, Joe and Tim individually, asking if they were happy for me to write our family's story. Each of them said the same thing.

'Yes, of course. I'm so proud of you.'

As a documentary-maker and ghostwriter, telling other people's stories has been the bread and butter of my career, but there has always been distance between subject and storyteller. Now they are one. Over the course of writing this book I've tussled with questions I still don't really have the answers to, like, is it ever okay to keep a secret? What is nature and what is nurture? What does anonymous mean today? And how do we create a meaningful life when we are longing for something we do not have?

Having answers is helpful, but making peace with uncertainty is okay too. I have now met all the men who 'made' me – Simon, Rodney and the two Johns. They could be an eighties punk-rock band: 'The Babymakers'. Excavating my existence over the past few years has quenched my curiosity and fortified my relationship with my family. I think we take things for granted less. I have learned that it doesn't really matter how sperm and egg meet, or even whose sperm and egg. What matters is the family they grow up in.

But while writing this book I have been living in a thick kind of grief that is hard to explain. I have written through seasons of shame, heartache and surrender, and, when attending writing retreats and my Master's course, I began writing alongside others who were doing the same. Courageous people writing their truths. Each experience has left me a little changed and a little more convinced of the power and importance of telling our stories.

Being held by the gentle hands of history has helped. My story rests on the bellies of those who went before me and it has been a privilege to tell some of their stories alongside mine. I realise now that the story of humanity is a story of fertility; they are one and the same.

My family tree is not simple; my lineage is not linear. It zigzags. Some of it has been erased, scribbled out by my parents and rewritten by me. My genes were borrowed, gifted from someone else's forest. And mine, to another. Family trees do not stand alone in the woods, sometimes they share resources underground. There are the branches we see and the roots we do not. Not all bloodlines flow with blood.

Stories like my family's have a happy ending: the children, the smiles, the matching dungarees. But there are the less picturesque memories that make up all relationships, especially those steered through hardship. No doubt there were disagreements; raised voices, frayed tempers and cold shoulders. But year after year, my parents had each other's backs; after they were told it would cost a lot of money, that they would need someone else's sperm and there was a 93 per cent chance it wouldn't work. In sickness and in health, in fertility or sterility. They had no children and then four under five at once. They stuck it out and in the end they got what they wanted, and perhaps a little of what they didn't; a daughter who grew up and accidentally threw a grenade into their agreement. A daughter who wanted to write about it and tell everyone so no one else would feel the same shame.

For my dad, who has struggled to tell his story, I hope there has been some comfort in his daughter articulating some of what he couldn't. I hope he knows how much I love him and that I'm proud of him too. He didn't have to agree to any of this: the IVF, the sperm donor, the book. But I'm glad he did.

In the tarot, the very first card is called the Fool. It depicts a man looking up at the sky as he walks off the edge of a cliff. He holds a white rose in his hand and a knapsack on his shoulder; everything he needs. The card is about trust – trusting that the universe will catch you, trusting that the path will unfold when the time is right. When the fool is deceived, he keeps on trusting. Despite being lied to or cheated, he carries on trusting time and time again. To an outsider, he might appear foolish.

When James left, I was pushed off a cliff, and my life as I knew it ended.

And then a new one began.

The truth is that in the eighteen months since my break-up, I've had one of the best years of my life. I explored Europe: Vienna with my sister, Paris with my half-sisters, Barcelona and Milan with friends. I went campervanning around Scotland. I started lifting weights and loving my body again. I competed in a triathlon. I camped at a music festival in a forest. I graduated from my MA with a distinction and a Dean's award. I left my career in television to work in a small independent bookshop in Yorkshire. I got the book deal of my dreams. I started feeling excited about life again.

And I also met someone. His name is Ollie. When I met Ollie, he was converting campervans – sawing wood and fitting new roofs – which reminded me of my dad. Now he's a personal trainer, empowering people to take control of their long-term health. Through nutrition and strength-building, he has helped me to improve my endometriosis symptoms, which feel more under control these days.

Ollie is thoughtful, hard-working and so achingly passionate about the people and things he cares about. He has been open and honest with me about mistakes he's made in previous relationships and from the day we met I have seen how much effort he puts in – through therapy, journalling, exercise, researching and reading – to become a better person every day. He inspires me, makes sure I eat enough protein and, most importantly, makes me feel loved and safe. He also shares a birthday with my grandma – the one with the Elvis photo – which my dad says is a good sign.

Three months into our relationship, I was complaining about my endo symptoms when Ollie floated the idea of me coming off the pill. I was surprised and delighted. He talks about our future children; their names, what sports they might do, how we might parent them together. It's something I've never experienced in a relationship before. My desire for a family was always something to be hidden and hardly mentioned. Ollie knows what I have been through and though, occasionally, a dark cloud of distrust rises up within me, causing me to spiral in fear, he understands and he stays. For the first time in six years, I have stopped worrying. I had been furiously pedalling a bike uphill on my own, but now it feels like I'm on a tandem bike, sharing the effort; finally able to look around and appreciate the scenery.

For now, getting pregnant still feels like a Sisyphean task, but I am hopeful. After ten months of trying, we've had no luck and are planning to start a fresh round of IVF soon. Despite my past, I know I have to keep on trusting people. Without trust, life loses its colour. The Fool is my favourite card.

Ollie has promised he will turn up on the day of the egg collection, and I believe him.

When I was seventeen, my English teacher introduced us to the poetry of T.S. Eliot and I was entranced; soaking up every word. His poems felt like puzzles, with multiple meanings to unlock.

There are a few lines from his *Four Quartets* series that get quoted often:

> We shall not cease from exploration
> And the end of all our exploring
> Will be to arrive where we started
> And know the place for the first time.

Professor Brian Cox used the poem to describe our relationship to Earth – the pale blue dot – in the age of space travel, allowing us to see it anew. But I think it applies to our ability to create life too. All the exploring, all the trial and error, has led us here, back to the place where we all started, sperm and egg, cells dividing. Becoming a parent is seeing the world through new eyes too, as if for the first time.

In the following, lesser-known, lines of the poem, I can't help but wonder if Eliot, who never had children, is talking about the spectre of infertility.

> Through the unknown, remembered gate
> When the last of earth left to discover
> Is that which was the beginning;
> At the source of the longest river
> The voice of the hidden waterfall
> And the children in the apple-tree
> Not known, because not looked for
> But heard, half-heard, in the stillness
> Between two waves of the sea.

Most books about infertility end with a baby. I know how stories work: they need a beginning, a middle and an end. Struggle, adversity and finally, success. The moral of these stories is that it's all worth it in the end when their little miracle is born. But this story does not end like that.

I'm still here, waving from the shoreline.

To all those people standing on the beach beside me, I see you. Please know that I am with you too, listening to our children, heard, half-heard, in the stillness between the waves.

Our stories are still being written, and there is hope between the lines.

Epilogue

Like yours, my life is still unfolding. I finished the book, but the plot continues and new characters keep appearing. Two months ago, I received an email alerting me to a new half-sibling DNA match. It was the first time in years that anyone had popped up.

Male, born in 1993, lives in London.

I saw he'd matched with Eliza too, as we were the only two siblings on that particular ancestry website. I imagined him clicking on the notification, puzzled by his results revealing two half-sisters, one in England, one in Russia. I sent him a message, introducing myself and letting him know that I was sperm-donor conceived, gently enquiring if that information was a surprise for him.

It was.

My chest tightened. I was dislodging a rock of something he'd considered certain his whole life. I pictured a cascade of confusion and questions pouring out of him while staring at a screen, hundreds of miles away. Someone else who had innocently wanted to know more about their family tree.

He knew he was conceived by IVF, he said, but not with a donor. I gave him some more basic information, careful not to overwhelm him, and tried to make him feel welcome in a club he had not intended to join.

I googled his name. He was the spitting image of the donor.

His replies were friendly and he thanked me for letting him know. He said he would speak to his loved ones and get back to me. I imagined him sitting down with his parents and having a conversation like I'd had with mine. A thirty-year-old secret abruptly uncovered by a stranger on the internet. How would they react? Would they come clean or feign a wrong result?

I told him to take his time and that I had more information if he wanted it, but there was no pressure to keep in touch. It was like having a conversation with myself six years earlier. Six years wiser and more weathered, I now feel able to support someone who, like me, had been climbing the branches of their family tree only to look down and see the trunk sawn in half.

Three weeks later my older brother, Tim, told me he had a new DNA match too. This time it was a first cousin on the biological father's side. She messaged him and was perplexed when Tim told her that he was donor-conceived. Eventually she concluded that one of her cousins must have been the donor, but she had no idea which one. Ever the technology-nerd, Tim used Chat GPT to narrow down the possibilities. A 95 per cent likelihood came up; it was the name of a lecturer of neuroscience, who had been teaching at the University of Nottingham during the time of Tim's conception. I texted my triplet brother, Joe. He had graduated from the University of Nottingham just two years before. His degree was in neuroscience. My heart raced. Could he have been taught by Tim's biological father?

Joe replied saying he didn't know the name. I searched further and discovered that, after three decades of teaching at the university, the lecturer had retired just two years before Joe started his course.

Around the same time, Sophie and Mary called me out of the blue. Sophie's six-week course of radiotherapy for her brain tumour had recently finished and she was staying with her mum in Nottingham while she recovered. A friend had called by the house and they wondered if I might be interested in talking to her. Her name was Helen and she was a former neighbour of theirs. Growing up, Zoe and Sophie had babysat her two children. Helen had been through early menopause in her thirties, so she and her partner, Torsten, used an egg donor to conceive their children, but had never told them. Now the children were both teenagers, they thought it was the right time to let them know. Of course I would talk to them, I said, and we set up a call.

Helen and Torsten seemed like lovely, normal parents who cared deeply about their children. Within a few minutes of the call Helen started crying. I could see she had the weight of the world on her shoulders. She told me she had been incredibly anxious about our call and about telling her kids, desperately worrying they might decide she wasn't their 'real' mum. I recognised the paralysis and the fear, the staggering enormity of it all. I talked to her about telling my siblings and how well they had taken it. How different it is to be intentionally told rather than accidentally finding out. As we talked through their fears and the different possibilities, I reassured them that it was the right thing to do.

'I actually think the person this will be hardest for is you, Helen,' I said. 'For my family, it's been hardest for my dad. I think the non-biological parent has to go through a kind of grieving process all over again. But I think it's really important that you try and do that yourself – in your own way and time – so it's not a case of your children having to look after you and manage that situation on top of their own, like I felt I had to.' Helen and Torsten nodded. 'They will have questions and it's important to keep the doors open for whatever they want to pursue in terms of their biology, without taking it as a personal affront to you as a parent.'

We talked about the nuances and complexities of anonymity. One of their children had been born before the UK law changed in 2005, while the other had been born afterwards. One child had a legal right to know details about their biological mother and the other did not. Helen cried some more and I could feel the years of pent-up emotion bursting out of her after keeping the secret for so long.

A few months later, Helen messaged me saying they had finally told their children the truth. They were surprisingly matter-of-fact and fine about it, she wrote.

'What's the problem? You're still our mum,' her son had said. His only complaint was that he'd have preferred them to use a donor with curly hair.

Speaking to Helen spurred me on to find out more about my own donated eggs. I had emailed the HFEA a year before, but their backlog was long and I was yet to receive a reply, so I decided to contact the clinic directly. The next day they emailed back. In 2022 my recipient had given birth to a baby girl.

Somewhere out there is a toddler, biologically related to me, but not mine. A little girl who was so wanted and will be so loved. I am delighted, though there is another emotion swirling in there too. I'm not sure I can name it – it's something between bittersweet and bereft. It is a feeling of things coming full circle and of the swooning, cyclical nature of life. I wonder at what age she might have the conversation with her family. I wonder if she will ever contact me.

A few days before I finished the manuscript of this book, my GP called to say that the NHS had rejected our appeal for IVF. Ollie and I had been referred, but because we had not been living together for more than two years, we didn't meet their criteria. A 'designated decision maker' had refused to even pass our case on to the panel since she believed it was 'not significantly different to others in the same position'. I was flummoxed. I didn't know anyone in the same situation as me. Who else qualified for IVF only to be abandoned by their partner midway through? They wouldn't even allow us to finish my previous cycle using my frozen eggs. We would have to sit and wait for another year to qualify. But when you're in your thirties with severe endometriosis and a low egg reserve, a year is a very long time. The other option was to pay for the IVF ourselves privately and thus revoke access to funding forever. As soon as you pay privately for a round of IVF, you are never allowed to access IVF on the NHS in the future, even if the private round fails.

After hundreds of pounds spent on repeat tests for me and a semen analysis for Ollie, the private clinic – the same clinic that treated me as an NHS patient – quoted us £9,000 for a single round of IVF. It was so much money. I thought of the years' worth of baby items we could buy; a pram, a cot, a car seat, clothes. All that money vanishing before the baby was even conceived. Conceived, if we were lucky.

I dug deeper and discovered that the clinic did offer a 'value' package, so long as you qualified. You must be under thirty-seven, I was thirty-three. You must have a body mass index of less than thirty, mine was twenty-one. And you must have a 'good ovarian reserve', but I did not. Despite donating ten eggs to a stranger just two years before and freezing six of my own, they did not class me as a 'good' candidate; my AMH was too low. The difference in cost, as a result, was six thousand pounds. There is a great injustice in the fact that the women who have the fewest eggs – the ones who need IVF the most urgently, who have the least time – are charged the most money.

When we set up an appointment to discuss our next steps, the consultant called Ollie by my ex's name. I was mortified. She was confused. She had not read my notes. I was forced to explain everything in detail, all while watching Ollie's dejected face reflecting back at me in the video stream.

'Ah yes, I remember you. I wondered what had happened,' she said.

No doubt I had been the talk of the clinic at the time. I felt another hot pulse of humiliation. A few minutes later the consultant logged on to her NHS computer and found the updated notes. When she realised her mistake she apologised profusely, but the damage was done. Logging off the call, Ollie looked sad and I was shaking. I told him I was so sorry and kissed his cheek, internally furious that this had happened. I was sick of explaining and repeating myself, letting people down and exhausted by more unnecessary hurdles appearing out of nowhere.

It was New Year's Eve when the GP called. 2025 was supposed to bring hope, but I felt punctured; deflated, sagging, shrunken. Ollie made Korean fried chicken from scratch and we had a quiet evening counting down the new year, just the two of us.

But I knew we had to make a decision. To pay or wait? I scrambled for other options. Since his interview for the book, I had kept in touch with Simon Fishel. As well as 'making' me in a Petri dish, he was also the founder of my local IVF clinic, though now retired. I told him my predicament and he suggested I look abroad instead, where IVF is more affordable. He put me in contact with a colleague who works with some reputable clinics in Prague. But since my book deadline was just days away, I resolved to start contacting them in a few weeks, hoping we could start a round of IVF by the spring.

Three days later I took a pregnancy test and it was positive.

I had never seen a positive test before, so I was hesitant to believe it. Day after day I tested again, seeing a stronger line each time. I was pregnant.

The cough syrup worked. Or perhaps it was the bad cold I'd

had during ovulation that month. Possibly Covid. My immune system was down, I figured, the cavalry were deployed elsewhere and the space invaders were not attacking the sperm for once. Or maybe it was all the positive changes I'd made during the year. The dietary overhaul, the strength training, the career change, the seed cycling, the microbiome tests. I will never know, but discovering – after years of trying – that I could conceive spontaneously was an enormous, overwhelming relief.

A couple of weeks later we went to my parents' house to tell my family. It felt surreal to say the words out loud. Everyone was over the moon. My dad opened a bottle of prosecco and we toasted. I had a sip then gave my glass away. All evening we laughed and we celebrated. I was so happy.

But in the middle of the night I was woken by an intense throbbing pain in my abdomen. I went to the toilet and when I got back I was in excruciating pain. I couldn't lie down and every time I moved it felt like I would vomit or faint. I begged Ollie to help me. The lower part of my pelvis was vibrating; searing and unbearable, and it wouldn't stop. Ollie helped me hobble back to the toilet where I briefly sat down before passing out. He caught me and I woke up feeling sick and disorientated. We headed back to bed and managed to fall asleep. The next morning I messaged my friend, Rebecca, who was also pregnant, to ask if what I'd experienced was a normal symptom of pregnancy, knowing that it wasn't. She suggested I go to hospital, in case it was ectopic.

I was seen very quickly in A&E. Blood and urine tests suggested everything was okay and I was referred for an ultrasound scan a few days later. That was the first time we saw the heartbeat. The baby was the size of a blueberry – a tiny embryo just a few weeks old, yolk sac still intact – in the right place, nestled in my womb. I held Ollie's hand and we both cried with relief. The pain, the doctors agreed, was likely due to scar tissue from my endometriosis tugging and pulling as my organs reconfigured themselves and the influx of hormones took hold. After a few more weeks of sudden cramps, the pain started to ease.

The week I found out I was pregnant was the same week I handed in the manuscript for this book. Part of me likes the poetic notion that I needed to get my story onto the page before I could start my new chapter as a mother. Or that these things happen when you're with the right person. That the universe conspires to make it all happen at the right time. But I don't really believe it. These things aren't helpful for people who continue to struggle with infertility. Did the universe decide that my parents were not ready? That they were incompatible? How could that be? My parents are the strongest team I know. Many people become pregnant in difficult and dangerous scenarios, where there is no love or poetry. There are some things we can't make sense of and I don't think it's always helpful to try to.

A few people have suggested that I got pregnant because I was about to start IVF again or because I'd stopped thinking about it or because I was less stressed. But I was in the final weeks of my book deadline, writing and thinking about infertility every day. I was feeling forlorn ahead of Christmas, childless, watching another year pass. I was researching IVF clinics, worried about how many rounds we'd be able to afford, as my friends posted pictures of their baby bumps online. I was all-consumed with infertility; stressed and suffocated by it. We like to fit things into our personal narratives of patterns and solutions, but the reality is that none of us really know the science and magic behind conceiving new life.

Ollie tells me I am much more calm and relaxed since being pregnant. The pressure has lifted; the crushing weight of infertility has evaporated overnight. Now it's just the weight of the eight-ounce foetus kicking around in my womb, reminding me they are there. Reminding me how lucky I am, for them and for Ollie. Being with him feels like a sturdiness that I have never experienced before. He is excited and energised by the prospect of being a dad, and he will be a brilliant one. Our potential as parents, and people, feels dense and abounding.

I was incredibly torn about writing this epilogue. It's not easy to read about 'happy endings' if you haven't had one yourself. Stories of spontaneous pregnancies and miracle babies may offer hope to those still in the trenches of infertility, but they can also feel like a kick in the womb when it seems that everyone else has their baby but you.

As I write this, I am eighteen weeks pregnant. My due date is exactly two years after my abandoned IVF cycle. My belly is rounding and my jeans no longer fit. I have become one of those women I envied, one of the stories I resented. Infertility had become a core part of my identity, so it feels strange and slightly embarrassing to be writing about becoming pregnant without intervention. But as my wise agent, Matilda, reminded me, we all have different journeys to parenthood and mine has certainly not been a straightforward one. Some people might conceive quickly but have a difficult pregnancy. Others may have a smooth pregnancy followed by a traumatic birth or postpartum depression. It's rare for anyone to have an easy ride at everything in life, especially when it comes to being a parent, so I'm trying to just be thankful, all the while still thinking about those who are struggling.

I don't have a baby in my arms yet, or a physical book, but all going well, the next six months should bring both. As a parent, and likewise as an author, I imagine you don't ever stop worrying, but for the first time in many years I feel content and at peace. Everything that was spilling out of me six years ago is now neatly folded back in. I have had my seams ripped open and sewn back up again. I feel softer and stronger. My life has expanded, and so has my definition of family.

Acknowledgements

First and foremost, thank you to my mum & dad, Ruth & Andy, Tim & Gina, Joe & Meghan. I feel so lucky to call you my family.

To Ollie, who wasn't scared off after our first date when I told him about the book I was writing. Your love and nourishment has kept me going through the ups and downs of writing, editing and pregnancy. I adore our little family and Rory is so lucky to have you as his dad.

To everyone who gave up their time and generously allowed me to tell their personal stories: Mary, Sophie, Zoe, Robert, John, Simon, Eliza, Libby, Lucy, Ben, Natalie, Alice, Roisin, Aisling, Louise, Ella, Holly, Dorothy, Hettie, Helen and Torsten. I am deeply grateful.

Thank you to the wonderful people at WME, especially my literary agent, Matilda Forbes Watson. From your very first email I knew that I'd found the right person to guide and champion my story. Thank you to Adela and Florence for all your support too.

To my brilliant editor, Michelle Kane, for believing in this book from the beginning and making sure it found the right home with the talented team at 4th Estate. Truly a dream come true. Thank you to Naomi and Iain for all your hard work and to Elizabeth Day – who I've admired from afar for many years – I feel so grateful to be part of the Big Day family.

Thank you to Sarah Stein at Harper and Erin Malone at WME in the US for believing this story could, and should, travel across the pond. Thank you to Gianluca Di Tommaso at NR edizioni for publishing in Italy.

To my half-siblings – Libby, Lucy, Ben, Eliza and Mike – we found ourselves on this bizarre journey together and your solidarity and humour have kept me sane (and laughing through the pain).

To Ruth, Rebecca M and Sufina – my first readers – for your endless encouragement and for always being so generous with your time.

To Rupal for your friendship and for whisking me away on beautiful writing retreats.

To the wombies and our remarkable three decades of friendship – BT touch!

To my excellent tutors at the University of Manchester: Horatio Clare, Jeanette Winterson, Beth Underdown, Kamila Shamsie and Ian McGuire. And to my fellow MA writers for sharing your work with such vulnerability and giving feedback graciously. Please keep writing.

To Emma and Tom for giving me somewhere to stay every week during my MA, and for your support when I needed it most.

To my long-time pal Millie Turner for my headshots and the endless creative and motivational chats.

To my friends Lucy, Gabby, Alex, Ella, Ally, Holly, Chloe, Suze, Cessie, Lewis, Anna Hall and the uni girls: Bang Tidy Barbarellas. Your cheerleading and support has meant so much to me throughout the years.

To Sara Sherwood and Kerry Ryan from Write Like a Grrrl whose workshops and retreats have been an affordable and life-changing sanctuary for writers like me.

To Ali Millar and Dan Richards for encouraging me in the early days, and to the Arvon Foundation for all the work you do to support new writers.

To Liz and Jonathan at Kemps bookshop for giving me a job where I get to indulge my passion for books all day and to my lovely and supportive colleagues Faye, Sam, Katie and Molly.

Thank you to Cheryl Strayed and Anna Whitehouse (Mother Pukka) for kindly allowing me to share your wise words and to Faber for permission to quote T.S. Eliot.

Thank you 'Rodney' for giving my siblings and I the opportunity to exist . . . and to all the egg, sperm and embryo donors who choose to help families like mine.

Finally, to all the researchers, scientists, nurses, doctors and campaigners who help people with endometriosis and/or infertility and take them seriously, thank you.